PHYSICIANS SHOULD TALK

HOW THE LOSS OF DIRECT COMMUNICATION IS KILLING OUR PATIENTS

E. Coy Irvin M.D.

All rights reserved. No part of this book may be reproduced, stored in a retrieval system, or transmitted in any form or by any means—electronic, mechanical, digital, photocopy, recording, or any other—except for brief quotations in printed reviews, without the prior permission of the author.

Copyright © 2018 by E. Coy Irvin M.D.

Loved (5.5x8.5) Self-Publishing Template © 2017 Renee Fisher
https://www.reneefisher.com

Cover Design: © TehsinGul - Pakistan

ISBN-13: 9781791933517

"Don't you doctors talk to each other?" In this book, Dr. Irvin calls out the elephant in every room where two or more physicians have gathered. To physicians: make this book the topic of your next CME or staff meeting. To the layperson: give this book to your doctor and don't return to her if she doesn't read it. What your doctor doesn't know can hurt you."

-Brian Jones, Principal Consultant, The Table Group

"Doing 'the right thing' is often difficult in our current world of healthcare. Thank you, Dr. Irvin, for broaching a difficult topic of how listening and hearing are two different activities. Coy's insight in his book, *Physicians Should Talk*, reminds its readers of the importance of removing ego and truly connecting with the patient's needs and concerns."

-Eli Pagonis, BS, MS, Founder and CEO, The Power of E4

"Dr. Irvin has written an important, thorough book on poor intra physician communication and how to fix it. He writes with a clear, concise style and is down to earth and practical in his suggestions. A must read for all doctors, particularly those practicing in hospitals."

-Stephen Imbeau, M.D.

Dedication

This book is dedicated to all the frustrated and tired physicians who have lived through the changes in the practice of medicine. Also to my wife Angie who made my medical journey possible.

Table of Contents

Introduction	9
Prologue	11
Chapter 1 – How Did We Get Here?	13
Chapter 2 – Loss of Autonomy	25
Chapter 3 – Fear the Call	37
Chapter 4 – Doctor to Doctor: Why Can't We Talk?	47
Chapter 5 – Doctor and Patient	57
Chapter 6 – Two Different Worlds	71
Chapter 7 – Whoa, Too Much Information	83
Chapter 8 – The Death of Professionalism	97
Chapter 9 – Everything Old is New Again	107
Epilogue	123
Notes	127
Acknowledgments	129
About the Author	130

Introduction

FOR MORE THAN 40 years, first as a practicing family physician and later as Chief Medical Officer of a large healthcare system, I have seen many changes in the practice of medicine. I grew up in a small southern town where the general practice doctors provided a full spectrum of medical care, from delivering babies to performing general surgery. I have seen the increased reliance on specialty care and the changes in family medicine introducing us to the now-infamous term, The Gatekeeper.

My undergraduate degree in business management gave me a different perspective when I attended medical school. My residency led me to family medicine and the development of a large family medicine group. My interest in lack of communication between physicians accelerated after a patient suffered a poor outcome due to a failure to communicate a test result in a timely manner.

I obtained an MBA and have spent the last several years working to help improve patient care and physician hospital alignment.

This book is an outgrowth of my experience and my work as a Chief Medical Officer and consultant. It will help shine a light on problems within our current health care system and how we can overcome many of those issues with simple, direct communication.

Prologue

WHILE WE WERE visiting a resort in the southeastern United States, my wife woke me at 4 a.m. in excruciating abdominal pain. The hotel staff quickly directed us to the local hospital emergency room. We unexpectedly found ourselves in a strange place in the middle of the night with a medical emergency. As a physician myself, the setting wasn't unfamiliar to me, but no one there knew who we were. We were just a patient in pain and her worried husband.

It took a long time for the emergency room physician to evaluate my wife and respond to her pain. Now, I know many patients come into the emergency room seeking narcotics, so emergency room physicians need to be cautious. However, erroneous first impressions can sometimes cause unnecessary delays in evaluation and treatment of real pain and acute medical conditions. Eventually, medical staff members began treating my wife's pain and evaluating her condition. We spent the next 12 hours in the emergency room, waiting for test results, a diagnosis, and a care plan.

The situation only became urgent to the medical staff after I revealed I was a physician and expected them to respond more appropriately. They ordered exploratory abdominal surgery, which was delayed because the radiologist and the surgeon were not communicating about what each one was looking for. This further delayed care and put my wife's life at risk.

Finally, at 11 a.m. the following night, after waiting for nearly 24 hours, physicians performed exploratory surgery and discovered a significant blockage in my wife's small intestine. Postoperatively she did well, and overall the care was appropriate. However, had the physicians talked earlier and clarified what each was looking for, the delay in evaluation, treatment, and surgery and the continued risk to my wife's life could have been avoided.

That experience brought me face to face with the firsthand realization that physicians should communicate directly with each other to provide the best care for the patient. Geography, facility size, existing policies, a patient's identity or connections, and other influencing factors shouldn't interfere with effective communication between physicians and among medical staff. This book is a direct outcome of that experience.

Chapter 1 – How Did We Get Here?

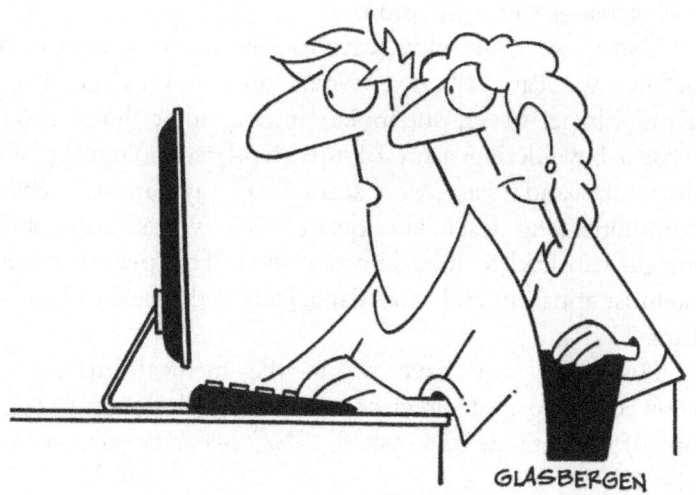

COMMUNICATION. WHEN IT works, we hardly notice it. When it's missing, things go wrong. And when it's missing in health care, it costs money, time, and sometimes lives. A brief look at the history of the practice of medicine reveals some interesting insights about what happened, and when, and what it means today.

* * * * *

From the time we're born, we communicate, first by body language, then by voice. We experience needs for the very first time, and we let them be known, often with great urgency.

It's really simple to communicate, right? All you have to do is *talk* and *listen*. In fact, communication is defined as the exchange of information.

Today, we have more ways to communicate than ever before. We can call, text, e-mail, instant message, Face Time, Skype, tweet, and poke, among other things. We have a bewildering array of tools and technology at our disposal, and yet we seem to say more while communicating less. The quantity of words, data, and images can lead to miscommunication. This problem may be most apparent and most dangerous in the field of health care.

How and why have we in the medical profession allowed the loss of direct communication between us? As one of my patients once asked, *"Don't you doctors talk to each other?"*

Often, the sad answer is a resounding "NO."

Thus, to paraphrase a famous movie line by Paul Newman in 1967's 'Cool Hand Luke,' what we have in today's practice of medicine is a failure to communicate.

Communication failures were a factor in 30 percent of the malpractice cases examined by CRICO Strategies[1], a research and analysis offshoot of the company that insures Harvard-affiliated hospitals. The cases included 1,744 deaths.[2]

Miscommunication among medical staff while transferring patients contributed to 80 percent of serious medical errors, according to one estimate by the Joint Commission, a group that sets safety standards and accredits health care organizations.[3]

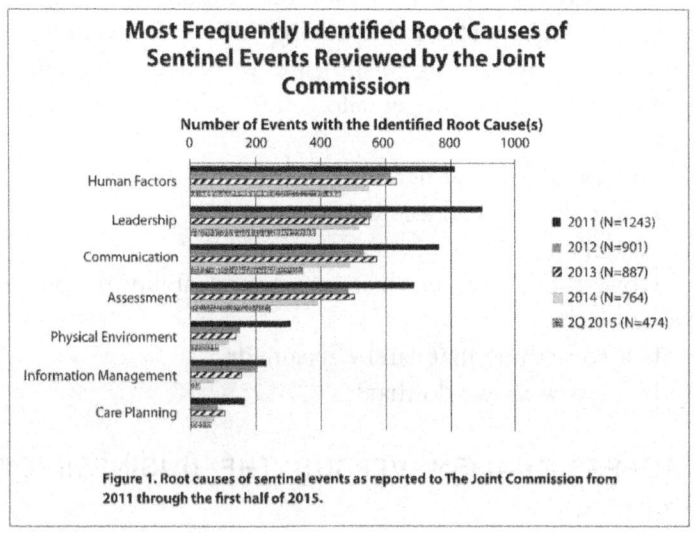

Figure 1.[4]

The Joint Commission, a nonprofit entity that audits, certifies, and accredits more than 20,000 health organizations and programs in the United States, has prioritized patient safety. Their studies reveal a clear correlation between lack of communication and serious patient harm. In fact, they have determined that miscommunication or lack of communication is a root cause of serious injury or death. As seen in Figure 1 above, the Joint Commission listed the leading causes of sentinel events leading to patient harm. The failure to communicate is a serious cause for patient harm.

Hospitals in this country waste more than $12 billion annually because of communication inefficiencies.[5] Annual medical malpractice payouts for communication breakdowns, including failing to share test results, more than quadrupled nationally between 1991 and 2012, to $91 million.[6]

To address this, the Joint Commission has set a national patient safety goal of improving the effectiveness of communication among healthcare providers. To put it simply, we can no longer allow this failure to harm our patients.

So how did we get here?

Has it always been this way?

Not likely.

How, then, have we lost our critical ability to talk to each other?

Is it something that can be regained?

If so, how do we do that?

Professionalism versus the Business of Medicine

According to merriam.webster.com[7], a 'profession' is defined as a calling requiring specialized knowledge and often long and intensive academic preparation. A 'business' is defined as any activity or enterprise entered into for profit. Based on those definitions, is the practice of medicine a profession or a business? To answer the question, let's look at a brief history of the practice of medicine.

THE BEGINNINGS OF MANAGED CARE[8]

Before the year 1900, most physicians practiced medicine in a single small office, much like today's cottage industries. However, in 1910, the first example of a health maintenance organization (HMO) emerged. The Western Clinic in Tacoma, Washington began to offer, through its own providers, a broad range of medical services in return for a premium payment of fifty cents per member per month. The program was available to local lumber mill owners and their employees. This was a very early example of prepayment for medical services or managed care, as it would later be called. This early example of an HMO did not become immediately popular with businesses or the American public.

In 1929, the Rural Farmer's Co-op Health Plan was launched in Elk City, Oklahoma. Farmers purchased shares for $50 each to raise capital for a new hospital, and in return they received medical care at a discount. The medical community opposed this new concept.

Also in 1929, Baylor Hospital in Texas agreed to provide approximately 1500 teachers with prepaid care at its hospital. This was the origin of the Blue Cross Blue Shield health care plan. Blue Cross Blue Shield has survived and become one of the major players in the insurance industry.

All these examples show the early influence of business practices on the profession of medicine. However, health insurance as we know it today is a relatively new concept in the history of American health care.

Further HMO development occurred in the 1930s and 40s around the time of World War II. Several HMOs were started then, and some remain in operation today.

- The Kaiser Construction Company started the Kaiser Foundation Health Plan in 1937.

- The Home Owners Loan Corporation organized a group into a health association in Washington, D.C. in 1937.
- New York City, seeking coverage for its employees, began the Health Insurance Plan of New York in 1944.
- In 1947, 400 Seattle families organized to form the Group Health Cooperative of Puget Sound.

As changes to health care swept across the country, many medical societies became concerned about the loss of professionalism in the practice of medicine. This led to the formation of early independent practice associations. The first one on record was created in 1954 when the San Joaquin Medical Society formed the Medical Foundation to compete with the Kaiser Foundation Health Plan. The Medical Foundation was an early adopter of the use of the relative value unit (RVU), which set the schedule for paying physicians. They also began monitoring the quality of health care received by their member patients.

Medicare and Medicaid

Some might say many of the problems we face now in practicing medicine began when politicians took an interest in how healthcare was delivered in the United States. As early as 1912, Teddy Roosevelt's Progressive Party campaigned on the issue of health insurance. However, due to World War I, progress on health insurance stalled. During the Great Depression in the 1930s, passage of the new Social Security Act did not include health insurance. In 1944, President Franklin Roosevelt outlined an economic 'Bill of Rights' that included the right to adequate medical care and the opportunity to achieve and enjoy good health. As a result of this along with the competition for workers during World War II, many employers began to offer health benefits, which gave rise to today's employer-based system. In 1946, the Hill-Burton Act paid for the construction of hospitals to close the healthcare gape in rural America. The Act helped rural patients have better access to medical care. Hospitals were required to provide a reasonable volume of charitable care as part of the Hill-Burton Act, which started the creep of government involvement into American healthcare delivery and payment.

In 1965, the most significant change to date occurred in the practice of medicine in the United States, when President Lyndon Johnson signed into law amendments to the Social Security Act, officially called "Health Insurance for the Aged Act: Old Age, Survivors, and Disability Insurance Act of 1965." Medicare and Medicaid laws changed how patients received care in the United States. Medicare provided health care coverage for older people, and Medicaid helped states pay for health care for citizens who were close to the federal assistance level.

Medicare fully inserted the United States government into delivering and paying for medical care. With Medicare and Medicaid payments coming directly from the government, patients were no longer responsible for the cost of and payment for much of their care. Removing this responsibility laid the groundwork for the unchallenged escalation of healthcare costs. By becoming the largest payer of medical care costs in our country, the United States government also became the de facto price setter for medical care.

In the 1960s, as the cost of medical care continued to skyrocket, the medical community found itself under enormous pressure to find a way to control costs. Because Medicare and Medicaid brought more patients into the market, the total cost to the government soared. Original estimates of the cost of Medicare and Medicaid were low; as it grew, costs of the programs were much higher than expected.

THE HEALTH MAINTENANCE ORGANIZATIONAL ACT

In 1973, then-President Richard Nixon signed the Health Maintenance Organizational Act as part of his national strategy to reduce health care costs. Initially, healthcare providers and patients made very little progress due to opposition. The 1980s continued the changes in healthcare as corporations began to integrate hospital systems, insurance companies, pharmacy companies and physicians into a business model based on controlling costs and increasing profits. Many hospitals began to consolidate with other hospitals, forming larger organizations in order to control their service areas. Hospital systems and medical corporations purchased physician practices. This produced many failed ventures, and introduced changes in how physicians and patients interacted.

The resurgence of managed care began in the early 1970s. 'Helpmate organizations' or prepaid health insurance plans began changing how physicians delivered care to patients. Managed-care companies were able to successfully shift the cost of providing insurance coverage from themselves to physicians and other providers. Corporations, seeing the need to control costs, aggressively promoted health maintenance organizations with their employees. The term 'gatekeeper' was coined to represent how primary care physicians would reduce costs by controlling the flow of patients to more expensive specialists and specialty care.

At the same time HMOs were pressuring doctors to do more with less time and trying to cut costs, other elements were escalating the cost of providing health care. The pharmaceutical industry realized significant profit and increased pressure on physicians by increasing the cost of drugs. When the pharmaceutical industry realized they could charge $100 or more a month for prescriptions, medication costs escalated at an astonishing rate.

In addition to higher pharmaceutical costs, the 1970s and 80s saw significant progress in medical imaging. The introduction of CT scanners and MRI machines drove the cost of care even higher. Other breakthrough medical devices added to the cost of health care.

Adding to the pressure on the system was a 1987 estimate by the Census Bureau of over 31 million Americans have no healthcare coverage.

Physicians generally representing only 5% of the cost of health care found themselves having to provide the best health care possible while maintaining very little control over the actual cost of that care. The HMOs were introduced as a way to try and control the costs as well as the perceived quality of care being delivered to patients.

This 'perfect storm' of cost increases mixed with lower reimbursement put patients and physicians at risk. The business of medicine had superseded professionalism, the downward spiral of communication among caregivers and the ultimate threat of harm to patients had begun.

HMO'S AND THE PHYSICIAN/PATIENT RELATIONSHIP

How much did the HMO concept influence the relationship between patients and physicians? Consider this: For many years, physicians enjoyed strong relationships with their patients. Patients and their doctors shared a bond because of the personal care the physician provided. Physicians felt patients respected and appreciated the unique doctor-patient relationship. This all changed when the concept of HMO coverage began to take hold.

As part of the HMO product, patients were no longer responsible for paying their physician. Instead, they paid a low co-pay at the time of their visit. In the early days, some co-pays were zero, some were two dollars, and some were five dollars. Competition for patients among the insurance companies accounted for the wide variability in co-pay amounts. However, something terrible happened. *Patients began leaving long-standing relationships with their physicians because they could pay a lower co-pay if they changed providers.* Doctors were shocked to learn the physician-patient relationship, which had always been at the heart of the practice of medicine, apparently meant so little to many patients. Physicians sadly learned the price of that relationship was as small as the five-dollar co-pay.

So how did physicians respond to pressure brought on them by the business practices of the insurance companies, the government and the employer groups, which were demanding low-cost care? They changed how they interacted with each other and with their patients. Physician reimbursement decreased just as the cost of running an office practice increased. It was the perfect storm facing physicians, and it placed them in an impossible situation. They had to see more patients in order to make a living.

Physicians sell time to their patients. With decreasing income and rising costs, they were pressured to do more in less time. This meant less time to talk with patients and other caregivers. Instead, they spent more time filling out insurance forms, getting permission to refer patients for care, and obtaining approval for medical tests. As demands on physicians' time increased, communication quantity and quality decreased. Unfortunately, patient care suffered. Why? Communication among caregivers diminished as physicians knew that no one in their profession had time to spare. They did not want to disturb each other, but in trying to be polite, physicians were putting patients at risk.

* * * * *

Over the next several chapters, we will explore the loss of autonomy and the many rules and regulations affecting the practice of medicine. We will look at how separation of inpatient and outpatient care has further led to a loss of communication. Finally, we will discuss how we can recover the lost art of communication so we can give our patients the best care possible.

Chapter 2 – Loss of Autonomy

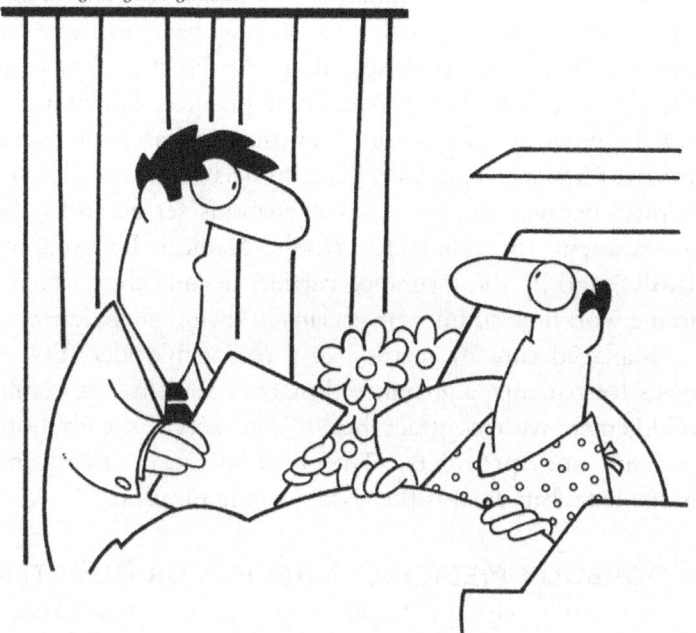

"Good news — your insurance company says you're feeling much better!"

HAVE YOU EVER felt like you were losing control of your world? How did you feel? Imagine you're a physician caring for a very sick patient who put their life in your hands. How would feeling like you're losing control affect you? How might it affect your patients and the care you're able to provide for them?

* * * * *

Physicians sell time. They sell time to their patients, to the hospital, and to insurance companies. If they spend more time on administrative issues, they have less time for direct patient care. With less time for direct patient care, there is a decrease in revenue to the practice. This is a loss for the practice, a decrease in revenue, and a cost increase for the physician's practice. The physician can feel a loss of control because the rules and regulations set down by the government (including Electronic Medical Records, or EMRs) and by the insurance carriers do not always factor in the workflow of busy physicians in their daily practice.

Managed care. It seems like a reasonable idea. Lower costs for patients, a guaranteed practice for physicians, and middlemen who contract health care services with both patients and providers. The benefits seem clear and immediate. But what is the cost? Communication.

COOKBOOK MEDICINE: A RECIPE FOR DISASTER

In the early days of health maintenance organizations (HMOs), payers required primary care physicians and specialists to get permission before doing almost anything for the patient. If physicians felt the patient needed a CT scan, they had to ask. If they felt the patient should have an MRI, they had to ask. If they felt the patient should see a specialist, the primary care physician would have to obtain permission from the insurance company first.

Now, you ask, who could give the necessary permission? Generally it was an administrative person with a book. The book contained an outline or recipe for how the patient or condition should be treated. Each HMO plan had its own recipe, or preferred course of treatment. If the physician's recommended treatment plan matched the book, the physician could obtain the permission needed to have the patient referred.

In the early days of HMOs, many 'cookbooks' were designed by the insurance companies with the goal of decreasing the cost of care, not necessarily improving the quality of it. Cookbooks were used to make decisions about which tests could be ordered, which procedures were approved, and when a referral was appropriate for the patient's condition. Physicians spent more time on medical record documentation, since this was how the insurer identified the plan of care and decided payment.

What happened when the cookbook and the recommended treatment plan didn't agree? Often the request for services or referral did not fit the book's recipe. Many times the plan in the cookbook and the physician's plan did not agree, causing significant frustration for the physician and the patient. In that case, the physician had to appeal the denied request. Avoiding the appeals process often meant tailoring treatment plans to the cookbook instead of the individual patient.

Physicians and their staff members were requested to leave direct patient care in order to handle the administrative burden placed on them by insurance carriers. This meant less time communicating directly with patients and more time spent getting the all-important administrative permission to do what was best for the patient. This took time away from patient care and started the micromanagement of physicians, leading to inevitable feelings of loss of control.

Caught in the Middle

Physicians slowly accepted the trend toward evidence-based medicine and managed care as 'best practice.' The development process endorsed by national medical specialties required increased documentation and those bothersome, time-consuming phone calls, again reducing patient and physician interaction. Many patients noticed their physicians were no longer staying in the room and talking with them, but were instead in a hurry to get in and out of the room and on to the next patient.

Physicians had to see more patients in order to address the increased overhead cost of managing patients through the HMO concept. Because physicians were paid on a capitated rate (a set fee per patient determined by an HMO regardless of the treatment required), they needed a large enough panel of patients to cover their overhead and make a reasonable return on their labor. In the business of medicine, where time equals money, any time taken away from patient care increased the cost of operation.

The concept of managed care in order to control cost is a good one. Using evidence-based medicine as a standard for practice is also a good concept, with the understanding that the evidence needs to be appropriate and vetted by physician specialties so that it is truly the best care for the patient. However, in the early days of cookbook medicine, much of the information had not been vetted or approved by the medical specialties, so physicians felt uncomfortable with the concept and the practice of cookbook medicine. The resulting loss of autonomy and decrease in time previously used for communication between the referring physician and the specialist began to take a toll on physician-patient communications. Because of the need to get a permission slip, or as it is really known, a referral number in order to refer patients, many specialists and primary care physicians began to talk less and less to each other, electing instead to talk through staff and the referral process set up by the HMO. This increased the risk of poor handoffs, loss of vital information, and patient harm.

Gatekeepers

With the advent of health maintenance organizations, another new word became common in the medical world. The term 'gatekeeper' became the new norm for patient care. A gate is designed to keep people in or out. The idea behind the gatekeeper model was to do more at the primary care level, where costs were lower. While this had some merit, it also resulted in many unintended consequences and work-arounds by physicians and their staff. Work-arounds were used to get patients treatment, medication, tests, or specialist appointments by going around the HML rules. This of course did not hold down the cost and frequently made treatment harder.

The plan allowed primary care physicians to address conditions that fell under the umbrella of primary care (family medicine, internal medicine, pediatrics, and obstetrics and gynecology). In theory, the primary care doctor would see patients and treat their problems without referring them elsewhere or requiring additional medical tests, thereby reducing costs. The noble goal of decreasing the cost of healthcare should have been obtainable. Initially, the gatekeeper approach was quite successful in lowering the rising cost of healthcare in the United States. Over time, however, primary care physicians realized the system would not allow them to send patients for specialty care or order tests they deemed appropriate and necessary. Even if they were able to get the referral approved, it took extra time and slowed down patient care.

Physicians also began to worry about their liability as patient care was managed. Would the cookbook be used in a medical liability lawsuit against them if the physician had chosen to deviate in their care of their patient? Also, the recipe might not work in every case and could expose the physician to more liability.

Patients felt the gatekeeper system was limiting their access to necessary care by denying the recommended tests or referrals. Their physician, who had always been their friend, their confidant and their healer, was now perceived as someone preventing them from getting a test or seeing a specialist. Patients began to see their primary care doctor as a gate or a roadblock keeping them from accessing healthcare specialists.

Physicians had very little time to explain to their patient why they were not going to give them a referral or order a test that the doctor felt was unnecessary. The capitated rate system meant they were paid a flat rate per patient in their panel no matter how much or how little care they required. There was little reimbursement for patient education. Many times, patient management took more time and effort than the system could support.

FOR WANT OF A PHONE CALL

Before the advent of referral authorizations, many physicians talked directly to each other about their shared patients. Primary care physicians and specialists would talk with each other about the shared plan for patient care. As communication between physicians decreased, the risk of patient harm and the loss of information led to many injuries and even patient deaths.

Consider the case of Mr. Smith (name changed to protect the patient's family), an elderly gentleman seen by his physician for an episode of chest pain. At the time of his visit, he was medically stable and had no acute complaints, but he did report a recent episode of chest discomfort while working in his yard.

His primary care physician had previously done a stress test on him and it had been considered normal by the cardiologist who read the test results. Mr. Smith's physician, however, felt he needed further testing and wanted a nuclear stress test done, which is a more specific test used to diagnose heart conditions. Mr. Smith had an HMO insurance plan that required a referral for the specialist to do the test and also required prior authorization for further testing should it be needed. The primary care physician obtained the authorization and referred Mr. Smith for a cardiac nuclear stress test with a cardiologist.

Mr. Smith had his test done and was not given any instructions except to go back to his primary care physician. His primary care physician had previously scheduled a follow-up appointment with him.

The nuclear stress test results were markedly abnormal, but instead of calling the primary care physician, as had been the usual practice and alerting him of Mr. Smith's potential danger, the cardiologist faxed the test results. The primary care physician's office did not receive the fax. This meant the patient and his primary care physician were not aware of the abnormal test results.

Unfortunately, prior to his follow-up appointment, Mr. Smith died of a heart attack.

When the primary care physician discussed the case with the cardiologist after the patient's death, the cardiologist commented that "because a referral number was needed for the catheterization and the number needed to be obtained by the primary care doctor, we (the cardiologist) sent the patient back to you (the primary care doctor) rather than just calling you and asking for approval to perform the catheterization on Mr. Smith."

This system failure that caused irreparable harm to Mr. Smith could have been completely avoided by a simple phone conversation between the cardiologist and the primary care physician. Prior to the advent of managed health care, the cardiologist would see a patient and perform the requested test. If the results were abnormal, the cardiologist would call the primary care physician directly and alert the physician about further treatment needed. There was no discussion of referral numbers – it was a matter of doing what was best for the patient.

As more and more administrative rules, obstacles and 'gates' are put in place, the focus on the system leads to less and less communication between physicians, in turn leading to avoidable patient harm.

In 2011, the Joint Commission patient safety goals specifically addressed the need for better communications in patient handoffs and in NPSG.02.03.01 the Joint Commission addressed the need for the reporting of critical results of tests and diagnostic procedures on a timely basis.

National Patient Safety Goal (NPSG) 2
Improve the effectiveness of communication among caregivers.

NPSG.02.03.01
Report critical results of tests and diagnostic procedures on a timely basis.

Figure 2.[1]

Grades

Another factor contributing to a growing sense of a loss of physician autonomy was the advent of grades and physician ratings. Again, this was a commendable idea, encouraging patients to evaluate and compare physicians and their care of patients. However, quality can be subjective, and difficult to measure. As we have seen before, unintended consequences could and did occur.

As the government and insurance carriers continued to address the need for better care at less cost, they determined 'grading' or rating physicians was a way to steer patients to physicians favored by insurance providers. If the 'best physicians' were chosen based on expert care and good outcomes, it would be hard to argue with the process. But as with any system designed to save money, there were winners and losers. Many physicians were graded not on the quality of care provided, but on the costs that were much easier to quantify. If they ordered more tests, made more referrals, saw patients more often, or used the hospital services more than other physicians, then they earned a lower rating *simply because they imposed more costs on the health care system*. This grade or ranking did influence patients' decisions about which physicians to see in their participating health plan. The rankings and grades also affected how insurance carriers paid physicians by using a bonus structure that gave more weight to the cost savings rather than the outcome of the care and the total cost of care. Finally, grading led to many physicians being removed from insurance plan panels, which meant they could not see patients participating in that particular insurance plan.

Unfortunately, physicians did not trust the intended use of physician grading. The lack of transparency on how the grades were determined made it impossible for physicians to trust the system. The system seemed to reward lower cost of treatment and not actual care outcomes. This reduced the feeling of autonomy for physicians, and continued to erode the physician-patient relationship.

Permission Slips

One of the most onerous and degrading parts of the early health care maintenance movement was the advent of what I like to call 'permission slips.' As discussed previously, ordering tests, placing patients in the hospital, and referring patients to other physicians for evaluation all required the use of referral numbers and permission slips. Each health plan had its own network of preferred providers. Many physicians felt this was an intrusion into their ability to take care of their patients by eliminating the use of their knowledge of local laboratory providers, hospitals, and specialists and what providers and services were best for their patients. The lack of transparency in how the network was developed added to physician skepticism. This process also caused problems for family physicians and internists by placing them in the difficult position of telling patients they could not have a test done or a particular medicine they might have preferred because it was not approved by their health plan. Many patients did not understand the rules of the HMO they signed up for.

Again, as a way to reduce the cost of medical care, the concept of managed care was and is a good idea. However, in the early days of managed care, many patients did not understand what they had agreed to, nor did they have a choice about employer-offered plans. Additionally, many physicians who signed contracts with HMOs did not read the contracts or fully understand what they had agreed to. In turn, this led to the sense of loss of autonomy by the physician as well as significant frustration on the part of the American public, causing the demise of many HMOs across the country. Currently, many insurance carriers have reinvented the HMO concept in the form of Preferred Provider Organizations or PPOs. PPOs allow more choice and decrease the use of the model of the primary care doctor being the gatekeeper, but the PPO continues to place significant administrative burdens on physicians and their staff.

Unintended Consequences

The advent of the HMO network as discussed narrowed the field of physicians available to see patients participating in the HMO plan. HMOs operated under a system of contracted physicians in their network. In order to attract patients, insurance companies wanted a large number of primary care physicians in their network, but they limited the number of participating specialists. Reducing the number of specialists disrupted many longtime referral relationships between physicians. Again, because physicians were forced to refer within the network, they often found that the network specialist was not appropriate for the particular situation, or they simply did not have a long-term relationship with the network specialist and did not know if the care provided by an unknown specialist was going to be best for their patients. This led to many in-network referrals being made, but no direct communication between the doctors. Physicians who had long-term referral patterns and relationships could no longer work together, and many long-standing physician referral relationships were lost.

This was an unintended consequence of designing the HMO system intended to control costs by limiting the number of in-network physicians. Since physicians were not allowed to refer outside the network, and choices within the network were limited, we again see a loss of physician independence. If patients did choose to go outside the HMO network and see a non-network specialist, their out-of-pocket cost would be higher. Many times physicians wanted to send patients to an out-of-network provider, but were not permitted to do so by the insurance carrier. Again, this increased physicians' sense of loss of autonomy.

* * * * *

In chapter 3, we will see how the delivery of medical care has changed, and how the loss of communication has developed. Let's look at how physician and nurse communication has changed, contributing to the risk of patient harm.

Chapter 3 – Fear the Call

©Glasbergen
glasbergen.com

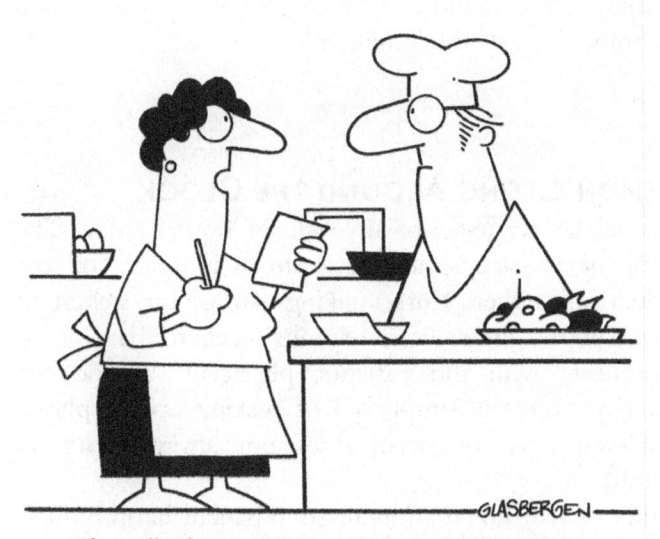

"The podiatrist wants jam on his toast, the psychiatrist wants nuts on his cereal, the plastic surgeon wants no wrinkles on her bacon, and the fertility doctor wants his eggs frozen."

WE'VE LOOKED AT what happens when physicians don't communicate effectively with each other. What happens when the lack of communication is between physicians and nursing staff? We conducted a survey among nursing staff, with noteworthy results that generated some practical solutions. In this chapter, we will discuss several instances of a breakdown in communication and how it can lead to patient harm.

According to Dr. Zeev Kain, during a typical hospital stay, the average surgery patient is shuttled between numerous departments, eventually seeing up to 27 different medical professionals. Ideally, the patient's records, medical history and treatment plan are shared seamlessly between the surgeons, anesthesiologists, nurses, and other medical staff who coordinate their care. ...Conservative estimates put the number of deaths related to medical error at more than 250,000 each year — and that number is likely much higher.[1]

* * * * *

COMMUNICATING AROUND THE CLOCK

As we all know, patients are sick 24 hours a day. The hospital never sleeps, and unfortunately many of the patients don't either. Nurses taking care of the sickest of the sick in the intensive care units need to be able to communicate with the patients' physicians around the clock. However, the simple act of picking up the phone and talking to a physician does not always work so smoothly.

Studies have shown an increase in patient harm both at night and on the weekends. In 2001, Bell et al. found that mortality was higher among patients admitted on weekends as compared to weekdays. Uneven staffing, lack of supervision, and fragmented care were cited as potential contributing factors. Similarly, Peberdy et al. in 2008 revealed that patients were less likely to survive a cardiac arrest if it occurred at night or on weekends, again attributed in part to fragmented patient care and understaffing.[2]

As Chief Medical Officer of a hospital, I noticed data indicating ICU communication and poor patient care was piqued when, as the CMO of the hospital, I noticed data indicating elderly patients were being moved to the intensive care unit in the early morning hours. After research, I realized these incidents were related to a lack of communication. Physicians, generally surgeons, had written orders with the goal of limiting after-hours phone calls from the intensive care unit. Each order was perfectly appropriate for the patient; however, the combination of orders was not. Physicians would order a medicine for sleep, a medicine for nausea, a medicine for pain, and a medicine for anxiety.

Each of these drugs, given separately, should have the appropriate result, but when they were given in combination, especially in a geriatric patient, respiratory arrest often resulted, and the patient was admitted to the intensive care unit and placed on a ventilator. After observing this, we talked with the medical staff about the dangers of stacking PRN orders. (PRN, Latin for pro re nata, means 'taken as needed.') The medical staff made adjustments, and the problem was eliminated. This generated concerns about delays in or complete failure to communicate with physicians about a patient's failing status.

In order to better understand these findings, we conducted a review of the data, which included feedback from the nursing staff. We asked several questions about calling the physicians after hours and why in many instances, calls to physicians were delayed or never made.

What we learned was surprising.

FEEDBACK FROM NURSES

The first question we asked: *"Are you afraid to call a physician about his or her patient after midnight?"*

Overwhelmingly, the nurses said they had a fear of calling some physicians due to the way they were treated when they called. Many physicians were polite, but some were hostile and even abusive on the phone. The nurses recognized the need to call a physician, but many times, if there was more than one physician on a patient's case, they called the one they felt was nicest on the phone and avoided the one they knew would be hostile. Unfortunately, the physician they called might not have the correct answer for the patient, depending on their specialty. So while the nurses could check the box on the form saying they contacted a physician, it might not be the best choice for the patient's condition and treatment.

Differences in training can result in differences in communication styles. Nurses are trained to relate information in a narrative format, which can conflict with a physician's concise, bullet-point approach.[3]

This is important because it can put patients in harm's way. It can also open physicians and hospitals up for liability issues.

The second question we asked: *"Do you ever stop calling if the physician has not responded in a timely manner?"*

The answer was 'yes.' The nurses reasoned they had tried several times to call a patient's physician and the physician had not called back. When asked further, they admitted using the same means and the same number each time, so if there was a problem with a phone number or the phone was not working, no one would know. Also, we noted the physicians would trade on-call status, but fail to notify the call center, so the nurses were actually calling the wrong physician. For example, one night when a trauma patient came to the ER, the general surgeon was called to care for the patient, who needed immediate surgery. There was a gunshot wound, which included a bladder injury, and the urologist on the call schedule could not be found. The surgeon repaired the problem, but felt consulting with the urologist would have been better patient care. Further investigation revealed the urologist had switched call status, but failed to notify the call center. This not only put the patient at risk, but left the surgeon alone and at risk as well.

Why is this important? Staff frustration can lead to reduced productivity. A study of communication between nurses and physicians in an urban hospital found that approximately 40 percent of the time that nurses spent communicating with physicians was "problematic time," in which they searched for contact information or attempted, but failed, to communicate with the correct provider (Dingley, et al., 2008).[4]

The third question we asked: *"When you need to call a physician in the early morning hours, do you delay the call and wait for the physician to round in the morning?"*

Again, many times the answer was 'yes.' The nurses would report delaying a call to avoid conflict with the physician. Our data and experience showed this could lead to patient harm. When asked about why the physician responded in a negative way to calls between 5 am and 8 am, the physician responded that calls during those hours were so close to a shift change that responding to them would be better directed to the doctor who would be on duty during the day.

This is important because a physician just coming on duty might not give an answer best suited for the patient's needs, possibly resulting in patient harm. Information can be inadvertently omitted or misinterpreted, leading to a progressive loss of information known as "funneling" and resulting in gaps in care or treatment.[5]

The final question we asked: *"When you call a physician to consult on the patient, does the physician come to see the patient in a timely manner?"*

The answer was 'not always.' Sometimes it might take more than 24 hours to complete a consultation. When asked whether they notified the original physician who requested the consult of the delay, the answer was that many times, they did not, giving another example of a failure to communicate.

Why is this important? When the attending physician sees an ICU patient and a consult is requested, it can mean the patient is deteriorating rapidly. Any delay in the consult being answered can potentially lead to patient harm or death. If the requesting physician does not know about the delay, a failure to communicate has occurred. If the need is acute, it is always best to communicate directly.

GETTING TO THE HEART OF THE ISSUES

After this discussion with the nurses, it was clear we had many issues to address.

- If physicians tended to be hostile on the phone, nurses would choose not to call them at all, not only leaving the patient in harm's way, but also leaving the physician and the hospital open for potential liability issues.
- When consulting physicians were delayed in taking care of the patient and the original physician was not notified, there was a delay in treatment and the potential for possible patient harm.
- When a physician other than the admitting physician was called, many times their answer to

the question was not the most appropriate for the patient's needs, and patient harm could occur.

When asked about why they were unpleasant when called at night, physicians spoke up.

- Many times they felt the call was unnecessary.
- Sometimes when nurses called, they were unprepared and did not have the information needed to answer the physicians' questions. (Incidentally, this has become more complicated as updating electronic medical records can delay care and generate many unnecessary phone calls.)
- Physicians complained nurses failed to call when there was a significant change in the patient's condition.
- Finally, physicians were frustrated when they were called and they were not on call.

When it comes to communication among caregivers, many variables are in play, including:

- The quantity of information
- The ever-changing nature of information
- The number of people tasked with carrying vital information forward (this relates to shift changes; the knowledge can leave with the person who's finishing their shift)
- The fact that not everyone knows everything that's important to be known about each patient
- An environment filled with interruptions. In fact, a study examining communication patterns among physicians and nurses found thirty one percent of communication exchanges involved

interruption, translating into roughly 11 interruptions an hour for physicians and nurses.[6]

What's the Solution?

These are not new complaints; they have been around for many years, with many attempts made to resolve them. Among those:

- Many community hospitals now have 24-hour intensivist coverage, so there is a physician always available in the hospital. It may be a pulmonologist, a board certified intensivist, or a nocturnist (a hospitalist who primarily works at night).

- For smaller hospitals or hospitals that have difficulty recruiting intensivists, there are now 24-hour Tele-ICU intensivist programs that use software to monitor patients so there is an early warning system for patients who are trending in the wrong direction. Physicians are available via the telemedicine system to answer concerns 24 hours a day. Many hospitals have seen improved retention of ICU-trained nurses, and have also used the tele-ICU to help teach younger nurses. This option seems to have improved the communication issue.

    Additionally, to address behavior issues associated with hostile physicians, many medical staffs have integrated 'Codes of Behavior' in their rules and regulations. These address the timeliness of consults, the timeliness of returning phone calls, and clarify the professional behavior standards expected of a member of the medical staff.

- Finally, there are programs available that outline what information nurses should have available when they call physicians. This includes having the patient's medical record available so nurses can inform physicians of any other orders given by other physicians, medications, allergies, and laboratory test results that might influence the physician's response to the question, assuring the correct information is communicated and the patient gets the proper care.

SBAR Sample

Originally developed by the United States Navy for use on nuclear submarines, SBAR is a simple safety tool that can help the nurse organize their thoughts to clearly and concisely relay information to another member of the health care team. Following SBAR, the nurse's conversation with a doctor might sound something like this:

S – Situation: Hi Doctor Jones, this is Joni on 4 West. I'm calling about your patient, Mrs. Smith in room 432.

B – Background: She's a 70 year old, second day post-op hip patient and has been complaining of intense pain tonight.

A – Assessment: She received all her scheduled antibiotics but started running a fever of 101 at midnight. Her incision is also quite red and I noted some new purulent drainage.

R – Recommendation: I'm concerned she may have an infection and I'd like you to see Mrs. Smith as soon as possible. In the meantime, I'm wondering if you'd like me to draw a CBC or blood cultures?

Figure 3.[7]

SBAR (Situation, Background, Assessment, and Recommendation) is a structured communication tool that standardizes communication between health professionals (Institute for Healthcare Improvement, 2011). It can be especially effective when a nurse is contacting a physician with a concern about a change in patient status. By clearly spelling out his or her concerns, observations, interpretation, and recommendations, the nurse using SBAR provides the physician with a more complete picture of the clinical situation than might be the case without the tool. In this way, the use of SBAR can prevent the scenario in which the physician underestimates the significance of a clinical finding conveyed via telephone.[8]

* * * * *

"What if?" What if the nurses and physicians came together and designed a system for communication, and what if they made the patient the center of their discussions? Physicians and nurses want the best care for their patients, and they sometimes get lost in the demands of the job. Addressing and improving poor communication habits can help us achieve what we all want: the best patient outcomes possible.

Chapter 4 – Doctor to Doctor: Why Can't We Talk?

©Glasbergen / glasbergen.com

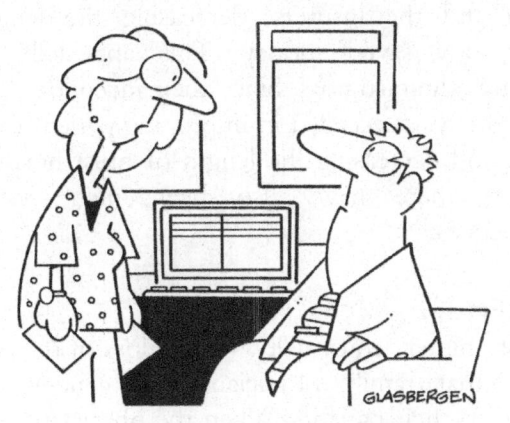

"The doctor will be in shortly to type on the computer and update your chart. If he has time, he will ask how you're feeling and take a look at your rash."

WE HAVE LOOKED at how the loss of autonomy and time has brought us to a place where physicians do not communicate effectively with each other, sometimes causing poor outcomes and patient injury. In this chapter, we'll examine several scenarios showing how physicians' failure to communicate continues to be one of the greatest barriers to outstanding medical care.

* * * * *

In the mid 1990's, hospitalist programs began to be introduced around the country. The idea was simple: full-time physicians in hospitals taking care of patients. The program's goal, promoted by managed care, was to cut the patient's length of stay and improve the quality of patient care. For the practicing physician in the community, not having to take an hour or more out of his or her day to make rounds on just one or two patients seemed to make great sense. The after-hours hospital calls and emergency room calls had always been seen as a burden. For the hospital and the insurers, decreasing the length of a hospital stay saved money. This appealed to many healthcare administrators. Since their inception, hospitalist programs have succeeded in improving patient care in the hospital and decreasing the length of most hospital stays. However, there have also been many unintended consequences.

Problem #1
The first unintended casualty was the loss of the continuity of care that family physicians and general internists provided to their patients. When the physicians no longer made rounds on their patients in the hospital, a disconnect occurred.

As this happened, the referral patterns between outpatient physicians and inpatient physicians changed.

Now, no longer does the surgeon know the referring physician on a personal level. Many outpatient physicians do not attend staff meetings or come to the doctor's workroom, where previously physicians interacted and got to know each other.

Loss of familiarity resulted in loss of communication. Hospitalists were now responsible for inpatient care as well as making sure the patient followed up after their hospital stay as an outpatient. Hospitalists also worked in shifts, so patients might end up being seen by several different hospitalists during their stay. This increased the number of patient handoffs, which increased the need for better communication at a time when there was less communication. In many instances, hospitalists did not understand their role as a referral source for the sub-specialty physicians. Hospitalists consulted many subspecialists during a patient's stay in the hospital, and many times they were not as familiar with the specialists and lacked a true understanding of the quality of medicine practiced by the specialists they consulted. Again, with primary care providers not coming to the hospital and not interacting with sub-specialty physicians, there was an increased risk for failure to communicate and the potential for patient harm.

Problem #2

The second unintended consequence was the patients' loss of the guidance from their primary care physician when they were in the hospital. In the past, the physician who knew them best also saw them in the hospital. Because patients knew and trusted their primary care provider, any referral physicians the primary care provider requested to see their patients were accepted by the patients because of their trust in their primary care provider and his or her judgment. The loss of the primary care physician from the hospital made it harder for patients to trust new, unfamiliar doctors. Communications became harder not only between physicians and patients, but also between physicians and referral physicians.

So you see how even something considered by most to be the way of the future -- the advent of the hospitalist movement -- added to the communication problems facing physicians.

Too Many Cooks

Let's see how the problems of the new practice model can affect patient care. Mrs. Williams was admitted to the acute care community hospital via the hospital's emergency room with onset of pneumonia, poorly controlled diabetes, and high blood pressure. She also complained of abdominal pain and difficulty with severe constipation. Mrs. Williams was taking approximately nine different medications, but wasn't sure what they were. Upon her arrival at the emergency room, the ER physician and nurses saw her and collected the information on her medications. The hospitalist admitted her to the hospital and proceeded to consult a pulmonologist for her lung problem, a gastroenterologist for her abdominal pain, and an endocrinologist to evaluate her diabetes. Now Mrs. Williams had four new physicians she had never seen before. Adding to the confusion was a hospitalist shift change, making a total of five physicians. Each one would come by her room and see her, but no one seemed to be in charge, according to Mrs. Williams. Each physician seemed most concerned only about his or her own area of expertise. Because the hospitalist had many other patients due to short staffing, they were unable to adequately oversee all of Mrs. Williams' care. This led to extra tests, medications interacting with each other in unintended ways, and a longer hospital stay for Mrs. Williams. Again, the lack of communication between all of the physicians led to poor medical treatment for Mrs. Williams and higher care costs.

DID YOU TALK TO DR. SMITH?

I believe the following story clearly illustrates how the loss of communication between doctors can cause great harm to the patient and disrupt the care we give our patients. As a Chief Medical Officer, I had to address issues occurring between physicians practicing on my hospital's staff. One particularly contentious argument between physicians came to my attention. I was told the surgeon and anesthesiologist had a significant argument while attending to an emergency room patient. Initially the patient had been seen in the emergency room by the general surgeon, who felt the patient did not have to go to surgery immediately. Since it was midnight, the surgeon felt the patient could wait for an early morning start the following day. However, the general surgeon received a report on the patient's CT scan indicating an acute problem and decided to go to surgery immediately. The anesthesiologist became irate, saying the surgeon only wanted to go to surgery immediately in order to protect the surgeon's existing schedule in the morning.

When asked if they talked with each other about the change in orders, the physicians involved said 'no.' The general surgeon said he told the nurse to tell the anesthesiologist of the change, but did not talk directly to the anesthesiologist. The anesthesiologist reported he was not given a reason for going to surgery immediately. When asked why they did not talk to each other directly, they both said there was not enough time. Eventually, they agreed the argument could have been avoided if they had

had a direct conversation. Again, the lack of direct communication led to misunderstandings, assumptions, and even to disruptive arguments, which in this case were avoidable.

I Didn't Want to Bother You

Several years ago, I was in my office seeing patients when my nurse came to me and said that Dr. Alan, a local cardiovascular surgeon, was on the phone and would like to talk with me. I excused myself from the patient I was seeing and went to talk to Dr. Alan. He told me he had just completed surgery on one of my patients and wanted me to know the patient was doing well and would be in the hospital for three more days. I thanked Dr. Alan for calling me and letting me know. Just before we hung up, he said, "You know, many of the doctors I call complain I am bothering them when I call to tell them about their patients." This made me very sad to realize physicians were under so much pressure to stay on time they did not have time to appreciate a call from a surgeon who had just completed an operation on one of their patients.

I've also had the opposite experience, where a physician admitted a patient of mine to the hospital and I was not informed. Since I went to the hospital daily for rounds, many times I would walk by the patient's room without even realizing they were there. However, the patient or their family did note I did not stop by and say hello, and this caused problems in our relationship. This could have been avoided by a simple phone call to let me know my patient, whom we both cared for, had been admitted to the hospital.

This has expanded exponentially over the last few years with the loss of communication between hospitalists and primary care physicians. It is not uncommon for a primary care physician to have one of their patients admitted to the hospital, treated, and released, and never know they were there. There are procedures in place to try and alleviate this problem, but it continues to be a difficult process to complete satisfactorily for both inpatient and outpatient physicians.

Ideally, the patient would come to the hospital with the primary care physician being notified by text, email or phone of their patient's admittance. Should there be a need to add to the patient's history or pass along information from the primary care doctor, then a phone call from the hospitalist to the primary care physician would be appropriate. And upon discharge, again an email, fax, text or even a phone call would let the primary care physician know the patient had been in the hospital and would follow up with them. This would be a much better way of completing the patient handoff.

Studies have shown that when the patient is seen within the first week of discharge from the hospital, they are much less likely to return to the hospital for readmission. Specifically, patients who have a clear understanding of their after-hospital care instructions, including how to take their medicines and when to make follow-up appointments, are 30 percent less likely to be readmitted or visit the emergency department than patients who lack this information, according to a study funded by the Agency for Healthcare Research and Quality (AHRQ) and published in the February 3, 2009, issue of the Annals of Internal Medicine.[1]

This has become extremely significant, as Medicare has begun penalizing hospitals for readmissions within the first 30 days post-discharge. Patient handoffs and the transfer of information are extremely important to protect the patient's health, prevent readmissions, and avoid patient harm.

Who is on First?

One of the most interesting failures to communicate between physicians has been the game of 'who is on call.' Many hospitals have purchased elaborate software is to try and track which doctor is on call for each of their attending physician groups each night. This can be a very difficult challenge, as many physicians change the call schedule almost daily. Call schedule changes to the master call schedule of a hospital have to be addressed so the emergency room physician knows who to call should one of the patients of a particular practice come to the hospital. This can lead to physicians being awakened in the middle of the night for calls they should not get. It can lead to patients being admitted to the hospitalist's service when they should be admitted to the primary care physician who still comes to the hospital. It also means patients might wait longer in the emergency room while the appropriate subspecialist is found to come in and see the patient. This not only leaves the patient at risk for harm due to delay in care, but also puts the other physicians on the case at risk if the appropriate subspecialist is not available to attend to the immediate needs of the patient in the emergency room or in surgery. Again, this is a liability issue and a patient care issue. The root of this problem is a failure to communicate.

The Future

With the advent of the hospitalist, we saw changes in how patients were cared for in the hospital. We saw a decrease in length of stay, but we had unintended consequences which in many instances, could lead to patient harm.

Now, in addition to hospitalists, we have intensivists for ICU care. We are seeing the development of pediatric hospitalists, neurology hospitalists, nocturnists, deliverists and trauma surgeon hospitalists.

* * * * *

The art and science of practicing medicine continues to evolve with pressure for new business models being pursued on a national level. In upcoming chapters, we will continue to explore how we can align physicians and hospitals better to deliver quality, cost effective care and improve caregiver communications.

Chapter 5 – Doctor and Patient

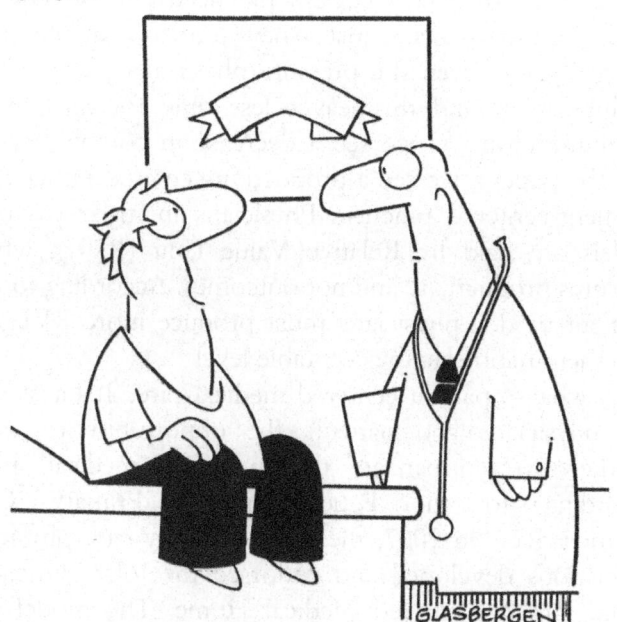

"I already diagnosed myself on the Internet. I'm only here for a second opinion."

IF OUR SHARED goal is the best possible patient care with the best possible outcomes, how do we accomplish that? In this chapter, we'll take a look at seven of the most common barriers to effective communication. We won't stop there – we'll look at possible solutions as well.

* * * * *

Let's look at a new (although some might say old) term, the trend to focus on patient-centered medical care. It sounds so simple and straightforward, doesn't it? Hasn't medical care always been about the patient? Many doctors would argue they have always practiced patient-centered medical care, so this is just a new term for an old style. Sadly, we have seen the pressure physicians are under to produce more and this leaves less time for meaningful communication. As we see a decrease in communication with the patient, we see a production-centered rather than a patient-centered practice. Physicians in many payment models are paid by Relative Value Unit (RVU), which measures productivity and not outcomes. According to this payment model, physicians must produce more RVUs to keep their income at an acceptable level.

So what is patient-centered medical care? It's a way to give physicians and patients the opportunity to work together to co-manage the patient's medical plan. According to the Patient-Centered Primary Care Collaborative, "in 2007, the major primary care physician associations developed and endorsed the Joint Principles of the Patient-Centered Medical Home. The model has since evolved, and today the PCPCC actively promotes the medical home as defined by the Agency for Healthcare Research and Quality (ARHQ).

"The medical home is best described as a model or philosophy of primary care that is patient-centered, comprehensive, team-based, coordinated, accessible, and focused on quality and safety. It has become a widely accepted model for how primary care should be organized and delivered throughout the health care system, and is a philosophy of health care delivery that encourages providers and care teams to meet patients where they are, from the most simple to the most complex conditions. It is a place where patients are treated with respect, dignity, and compassion, and enable strong and trusting relationships with providers and staff. Above all, the medical home is not a final destination. Instead, it is a model for achieving primary care excellence so that care is received in the right place, at the right time, and in the manner that best suits a patient's needs."[1]

The Medical Home model puts the patient's needs at the center of each encounter by having a team approach to care. In order to have the patient more involved in making decisions about the medical care offered by the physician, there must be clear communication between the doctor and patient, and time for the patient to understand their options. Patients need the information necessary to make good decisions about their treatment plans. Physicians must relay to the patient the options for treatment, and give them both the benefits of the treatment as well as any negative consequences that might be associated with each treatment option. In our RVU world of production, taking the time to thoroughly explain each option unfortunately increases the cost of the care and in many instances decreases what the physician will be paid for the patient encounter.

As we move forward with patient-centered medical care and patient-centered medical homes, we need to value physicians' time and pay them accordingly. The move to value-based purchasing is a start in the right direction, but going from a fee-based service to a quality-rewarded service will take time and potentially cause great disruption in the system. Many have suggested it is akin to having one foot in the boat and one on the dock. Catastrophe could happen at any moment. There must be a bridge between payment system changes to allow for the cost of data collection and reporting as well as the infrastructure needed to make the change. MACRA (Medicine Access and Chip Reauthorization Act of 2015), the proposed new system, will take much time and money to implement and the payers must help with the conversion. Under MACRA, participating providers are paid based on the quality and effectiveness of the care they provide.[2]

At a time when the need for medical care and specifically more physicians is growing, instead of freeing up physician time from non-value tasks like data entry and data reporting, we continue to place on physicians tasks which take away time from the valuable patient interaction. The introduction of the electronic medical record, the ICD 10 system (an updated coding system for physicians to use in patient billing, increasing the number of codes from 16,000 to 70,000, adding more specificity but taking more time and making correct billing a more difficult task for physicians), the idea of value-based purchasing, and the demands of increased documentation all take time away from what physicians value the most – his or her time with patients and the ability to give patients the best medical care with the best outcomes.

ROAD BLOCKS TO BEST CARE

What are some of the roadblocks that prevent physicians from communicating effectively with their patients?

- *Medical jargon* – the use of medical jargon can confuse a patient so they do not really understand what is going on with their health.

- *Fear* – the patient is fearful of what might happen to them and cannot really grasp what the physician is saying to them.
- *Cultural differences* – the conversation does not translate due to a failure by the physician to understand where the patient comes from and how they see the world.
- *Bedside manner* – the physician fails to relate to the patient because of how they present themselves.
- *Education differences* – the physician talks at a level the patient may not be able to understand.
- *Time* – time pressures do not allow for good explanations of the patient's condition.
- *Lack of follow through* – failure to ask if the patient understands, and/or a failure to answer the patient's questions.

Jargon – Or How We Get Lost in Translation

Let's look at an example of how medical jargon can affect the patient experience.

Mrs. Smith comes to her doctor complaining of her heart 'jumping and bumping.' The physician takes her history and does a physical exam. Next, the physician tells the patient she has palpitations, which could be related to an irregularity of her heart. He explains it could be atrial fibrillation, PVCs, or a disorder of her mitral valve. Mrs. Smith is confused and possibly frightened, but the physician feels she has received a clear explanation about the possible causes of her palpitations. Knowing the problem can be treated easily, the physician is not concerned, but Mrs. Smith does not understand any of the terms used. When she receives a prescription for a beta-blocker, which should slow her heart rate, she is even more confused and concerned when the physician tells her about the many side effects she could experience.

So what went wrong? The physician feels he has given the patient the information she needed. Mrs. Smith feels confused, scared, and totally dissatisfied with the physician's explanation. Neither knows what the other is thinking. Ultimately, Mrs. Smith leaves, does not fill the prescription, and continues to suffer from heart palpitations. The physician goes on to see the next patient feeling satisfied he has treated Mrs. Smith appropriately. Thus through the use of correct but undefined medical terms (jargon), we see a failure to communicate and the ultimate failure of the treatment plan.

How do we improve the previous scenario? As with most communication issues, it takes time to clearly explain unfamiliar terms. Upon hearing the words 'PVC' and 'atrial fibrillation,' Mrs. Smith should have stopped the physician and asked questions about her real concerns, such as "What do these terms mean? Am I in danger? Am I going to have a heart attack? Could I die and leave my family?" Likewise, the physician could stop and ask Mrs. Smith if she understood what they had discussed. The physician could use the read-back technique and have Mrs. Smith explain in her own terms what she understood about the discussion so the doctor would know she understood what had been said. This would better address the lack of understanding and likely improve the transfer of information.

Medical advances and new medications generate more terms and medical jargon that take time to explain. Physicians who are already under pressure to see more patients often struggle to find the time to explain medical terms to the patient, who is the one most affected by the conditions, treatments, and medications which need to be discussed.

Fear

Some of the terms used in a physician's daily work setting seem normal and routine. But to the patient, they are anything but normal and routine. For instance, Mrs. Jackson sees her physician to follow up on results of a recent lung cancer screening test. She has a long history of smoking and is very aware that her smoking can lead to illness, so she worries about what the doctor will say. As the doctor starts to explain the test findings, Mrs. Jackson is already nervous and worried. The doctor explains a *mass was found on her scan in her lungs,* and further explains the mass could be benign or it could be a cancer. At this point Mrs. Jackson *has heard the dreaded 'C' word* and from now until the end of the appointment, she does not hear anything else the physician says to her because she feels like she has been given a death sentence. To add to her difficulties, follow-up testing will require referral to a surgeon for a biopsy which will take up to two weeks, so Mrs. Jackson must live with her uncertainty and her dread for 14 days. It seems the system and the use of the term 'cancer' has devastated Mrs. Jackson and her outlook on life. How could this have been avoided? What should the physician have done differently to really communicate with Mrs. Jackson?

Whenever we use terms like 'cancer,' it is essential that we understand *how they will be received by the patient.* It is important that we plan ahead for such encounters and do a few simple things to make sure the patient not only receives the correct information, but also receives it in a way that ensures clear communication. The physician could have suggested Mrs. Jackson bring along a supportive person to help her clearly hear the results of the test and what the possible next steps and alternatives might be. This could help give her necessary support and possibly lessen the shock of hearing the term 'cancer.' It would also give Mrs. Jackson someone who clearly and objectively heard what the plan and discussion was after the term 'cancer' was used.

It is also helpful to have other members of the healthcare team work closely with the patient and address any fears or issues they might have. Treating the patient and understanding things from their point of view is vital to addressing their concerns. This concern for the whole spectrum of patient care affects the patient's overall impression of the health care they are receiving. Especially helpful is the ability to engage the patient as a vital part of the treatment plan – things aren't just happening to them; instead, they are vital, active participants in their own ongoing care.

Finally, it is important for the physician to be sure Mrs. Jackson understands what her options are, what the treatment plan will be, and possibly what the risks versus benefits of the treatment are. The physician can self-check to ensure good communication by asking her to explain her understanding, and address her concerns about their discussion by using open-ended questions like "Do you understand what we are going to do next?" Providing and briefly reviewing clear written instructions will also help lessen the risk of incomplete or ineffective communications. Remember, any handouts provided should be written at a grade level appropriate for the patient's understanding.

CULTURAL DIFFERENCES

As the need for physicians has grown in the United States, we've seen growth in the number of non-US trained medical doctors helping fill the gap. We have also seen an increase in immigration, generating more patients with different cultural backgrounds. This can lead to more communication challenges between the physicians and patients. In some instances, background and cultural differences between physicians and patients have led to patient harm. Using terms like 'positive' and 'negative' can be perceived in different ways, unintentionally communicating the wrong outcome. Language challenges between physicians and non-English speaking patients can and do cause harm because of incomplete communication. Misunderstanding symptoms and concerns patients bring to the visit can lead the physician to make the wrong diagnosis and cause the patient to fail to understand the treatment plan. The opposite can also lead to problems: think about the physician from another country and culture who is challenged every day with understanding varied regional cultures, accents, and local word usage. Imagine being from India and trying to understand a south Texas drawl and the meaning of words such as 'fixin' and 'hogwash.'

Bedside Manner

A physician's bedside manner can be a major stumbling block to patients following physicians' instructions. 'Bedside manner' is a term used to refer to the demeanor with which a physician interacts with his or her patients. There are many gifted physicians who use empathy and have a high self-awareness, allowing them to address patient concerns in a way that builds the patient's confidence in the physician's advice. They would score well on the emotional intelligence scale.

Doctors tend to learn their style of bedside manner by observing other physicians whom they see as role models. Being able to empathize with the patient and clearly convey a sense of caring is extremely important to not only establishing good communication, but also encouraging the patient to follow the medical plan.

EDUCATION

Another factor contributing to effective communication is the discrepancy in education levels between patient and physician. Many times, patients are unable to understand what the physician is telling them due to their level of education. Because many patients read at a below-average level, when they interact with their physician, there can be a failure to communicate effectively.

There are two relatively simple ways to address this issue. The first way is for the physician to ascertain the patient's level of understanding early in the relationship and then try and put the discussion in a framework that the patient can understand. Using the read-back method, a physician can have the patient explain what was said to them. If the patient does not repeat the plan back correctly, the physician can further clarify things with the patient.

The second way to improve the communication is for the patient to bring a surrogate or objective go-between to the appointment so that the information provided by the physician is heard by two people, thus improving the chances of clear communication. For instance, a grandson comes with his grandmother to be sure she knows what to do when they leave.

TIME

The dilemma of the patient failing to get a medical screening test as ordered by the physician can also lead to a poor medical outcome. For example, a patient comes to the office for a preventative screening physical and is scheduled to have a colonoscopy. A colonoscopy is an evaluation of the gastrointestinal tract, and unfortunately requires the patient to do a great deal of physical preparation. Patients may have many concerns and misunderstandings about the process of preparing for a colonoscopy. There also is a cost involved in the screening test, which can be a barrier to patient compliance. Many times a large copayment is required, or the patient's insurance company does not cover the cost of the screening test. All these reasons can cause the patient not to get the test done. It is important for the physician to clearly relate to the patient the process for preparing for a colonoscopy. It is equally important that the physician listens to the patient's concerns and addresses them in order to improve patient adherence to the advice and ultimately have the patient get the screening test done. The physician needs to fully explain both the importance of the test and the risk to the patient. Again, this takes time. It may be best to use other members of the care team to answer all of the patient's questions before the procedure and follow up with the patient after the test is completed.

LACK OF FOLLOW THROUGH

Why would a patient see a doctor and then not follow the physician's advice? Recent studies have suggested patients only fill 30% of the prescriptions given to them by their doctor.[3] Further, the number of missed appointments and the failure by patients to keep follow-up appointments continues to be an issue in the day-to-day care of the patient.

For the best care and a healthy patient, it is important to have good medication adherence and for the patient to keep follow-up appointments. When patients do not fill their prescriptions or do not go for preventive testing such as a mammogram or a colonoscopy, their medical care is not complete, increasing the likelihood of illness in the future.

If we are truly to be effective as physicians, we must communicate the importance of medications, especially when considering the cost of medications and the difficulty in taking a daily medicine. As physicians, we often feel the patient should be able to remember to take their medications as directed. It is not until we begin to take medicines on a daily basis ourselves that we realize how difficult it is to accurately take medicine as prescribed. We must communicate better to our patients about the need for medications, especially those for asymptomatic conditions like hyperlipidemia and hypertension.

Other factors contribute to patients not filling their prescriptions. Sometimes the cost of medicine prohibits a patient from buying it. Sometimes the patient forgets to fill the prescription. However, the number one reason for the patient not filling a prescription is *a lack of understanding of the need for and importance of the medication.* This falls squarely on the shoulders of the physician for failing to communicate to the patient the importance of taking the medication as well as its benefits and potential risks. Because the problem is so prevalent, many insurance companies, hospitals, and physician offices have begun to track whether or not the patient filled a prescription and if the prescription is being refilled in a timely manner. If those things are not being done, then the patient receives a phone call from the doctor's office or the hospital or the insurance company to discuss why they are not taking their medication as prescribed. Questions that would be best directed to the physician now fall on the ears of the insurance company representative – not the best way to communicate.

Finally, the incidence of missed appointments by patients and failure to follow up can cause great harm and damage to the patient and can increase liability risk for the physician. Many times in a busy physician's office, a patient will be sent for a test that comes back to the office with a positive result. It is important for the patient to return to the office and review the medical report to determine what, if any, further actions are needed. If a patient fails to attend the appointment, many times this can cause a delay in treatment and can lead to harm to the patient. Having built-in systems for tracking missed appointments and bringing the patient back to the office is extremely important. There are now many companies offering software and services to help patients and physicians make appointments and reschedule missed appointments. By adding an extra layer of review, a physician can avoid missing patient follow-up and prevent possible harm to the patient.

OVERCOMING ROADBLOCKS TO COMMUNICATION

As we have discussed the need for better communication between physicians and patients, we cannot overstate the importance of documenting all encounters with the patient not only in the office but also by telephone, text, mail, or other social media. It is essential for physicians to document their interactions with patients not only to prevent liability issues, but also to be able to determine when patients fail to follow instructions given to them. As physicians, our goal is to address the concerns of our patients and give them the best health care possible. To the extent possible, we need to communicate properly with them so they understand the importance of following the plan for their medical care. It is also important we take into consideration their unique concerns and address them, giving them options which allow them to make educated choices about the type of care they want and the outcomes they wish to obtain (patient centered care). Cultural differences, language barriers, the use of medical jargon, and the lack of time all pose barriers to effective communication and can lead to poor communication.

* * * * *

These point to the inevitable question: *how can we do a better job communicating with our patients?* Will the payment system support the changes we need to make in order to communicate more effectively, and will value-based purchasing help us improve? Only time will tell if we can change the system so physicians and patients can communicate effectively.

Chapter 6 – Two Different Worlds

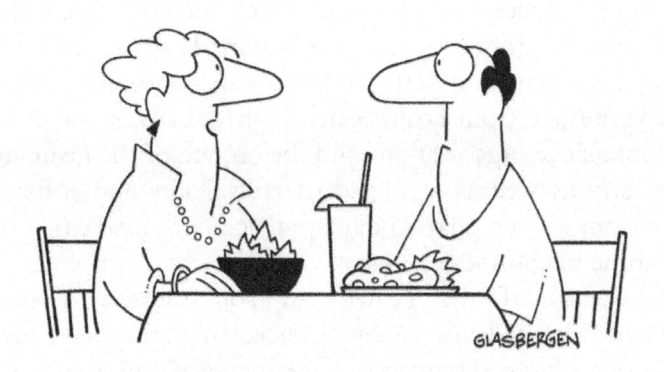

"When I'm dieting, my doctor says it's OK to cheat once a week. I'm going out with your friend Larry tonight."

THE PRACTICE OF medicine vs. the business of health care. From a cottage industry with sole physicians and independent community hospitals, medicine has grown into a business that is one of the country's largest economic sectors. Is it any surprise physicians can occupy two different worlds? Here's a look at how to close the communication gap, including a practical list of rules of communication engagement.

* * * * *

The Business of Health Care

With the proliferation of mergers among hospitals and the development of corporate medicine with large medical groups, it's not surprising that drugstore chains are opening clinics and hospitals are opening drugstores. Major food producers now invest in medical care, and even the retail giant Wal-Mart can't pass up the opportunity to make money from health care. With the advent of health maintenance organizations and the growth of the insurance industry as well as a myriad of consultants and software companies, the day-to-day practice of medicine has become big business.

Because of the growth of sophisticated business practices in medicine, many physicians feel they have been left out of the discussion. It seems as if physicians and administrators live in two completely different worlds.

Who's Getting it Right?

There are bright spots like the Mayo Clinic and the Cleveland Clinic where physicians in leadership positions are working hard to close the communication gap between administrators and physicians.

Many insurance companies are hiring physicians to not only do medical reviews, but also to fill positions of leadership to help address the great divide between physicians and the business practices of the company. Still, the goal of good communication and true alignment eludes us. Why is this a problem, and can it ever be overcome? Let's explore further.

PRACTICE VS. BUSINESS

As a chief medical officer for a major health care system, I had a unique perspective on both sides of the great divide. Physicians would often marvel at the actions of the administration and ask why they did what they did. At the same time, administrators would question why physicians did what they did. While both sides wanted to provide the best healthcare possible for patients, the failure to communicate prevented alignment and kept both sides from addressing the issues challenging both physicians and hospital administrators.

'Physician alignment' has become the catchphrase of the day, and many hospital administrators have mistakenly decided the best way to align physicians is to employ them. Many physicians, tired of dealing with the day-to-day problems of running a practice and the burden of ever more mandates coming from Washington, have chosen to become employed. (Physicians call it a practice, and administrators call it a business.) The ever-climbing cost of operating the physician practice and the implementation of the electronic medical record as well as the changing payment systems have all profoundly influenced the migration of physicians from private practice to an employment arrangement.

An Ever-Widening Gap

Physician burnout coupled with frustration over continued mandates have widened the gap between administration and the medical staff at many institutions. Mandates include:

- Meaningful Use. "Under the Health Information Technology for Economic and Clinical Health (HITECH Act), which was enacted under the American Recovery and Reinvestment Act of 2009 (Recovery Act), incentive payments are available to eligible professionals (EPs) who successfully demonstrate meaningful use of certified EHR technology. The Recovery Act specifies three main components of meaningful use: The use of a certified EHR in a meaningful manner, the use of certified EHR technology for electronic exchange of health information to improve quality of health care and the use of certified EHR technology to submit clinical quality and other measures."[1]
- HCAPS. "Hospital Consumer Assessment of Healthcare Providers and Systems, an instrument to measure patient perceptions of care to provide consumers with information that might be helpful in choosing a hospital."[2]
- Star Ratings. "The US Centers for Medicare and Medicaid Services (CMS) released the first ratings list for the Medicare Overall Hospital Star Ratings Program on July 27, 2016. CMS developed the program to help consumers make more informed decisions by giving them a way to compare hospitals based on quality ratings."[3]

The need for both the medical staff and hospital administration to share common goals – alignment – is of utmost importance and can make all the difference in providing outstanding medical care and delivering good patient outcomes. In this chapter we will discuss a few stories showing the gap between hospital administration and physicians.

ADMINISTRATORS DO THE STRANGEST THINGS

As a chief medical officer and consultant, I have always been interested to see how far apart physicians and administrators really are when they feel good communication has occurred. Let's start by telling a story which occurred in a large university medical center in the northeast. I refer to it as the *'Big Hole.'*

Medical university administrators felt it was time to build new offices for the medical school faculty, and they had a few conversations about the building with different faculty members, which they assumed meant it was okay to proceed. The university purchased land next to the hospital and invested in architectural drawings. They even began the initial site work for the new buildings by digging a large hole. Then the university administration brought the faculty members and department chiefs together to discuss the new building. After the meeting, administrators sent out an email to all faculty members announcing the agreement to build the building and going so far as to say the chiefs of each department had signed on.

Shortly after this email went out, the head of the medical school faculty sent an email in which he complained the building was a surprise; they had not agreed to the new office building. The project collapsed, and further distrust developed between the administration and the physicians. Currently, there is a nice and expensive parking garage sitting where this building was to be built.

How is it possible for millions of dollars to be spent on a project to house the medical staff offices without a clear agreement from the medical staff to occupy the offices? Many times in the process of trying to communicate a message between administrators and physicians, there is a failure. This happens because physicians are busy. Relying on indirect communication methods like faxed announcements, emails or letters will not get the message across. There must be direct communication. As you can see from this story, not communicating directly can be a very expensive lesson.

As physicians continue to have less and less time to read emails and letters and attend meetings because of the needs of their patients and the demands of maintaining electronic medical records, we are faced with an ever-growing challenge to successfully communicate with physicians. Effective communication not only helps avoid expensive failed projects, but it helps prevent poor alignment of the medical staff and administration. Good effective communication can and should lead to physician buy-in and alignment of both the physicians and the health system.

NINE TIMES NINE

There is an old saying about how to communicate with medical staffs. In order to successfully communicate with medical staffs, many administrators feel you must communicate nine different ways and do it nine times. Many administrators send out emails, schedule meetings, and conduct hallway discussions, and they feel the message has successfully gotten to the practicing physician. However, because of time constraints and differing priorities of the medical staff, good attempts at communicating can fail. Part of the problem lies in misunderstandings on each side. In order to communicate clearly and successfully, one must have a good understanding of *whom,* *why,* and *what* they are communicating to the other party. This failure has happened many times in the past, when administrators make incorrect assumptions about physicians based on their own past experience. The same can be said for physicians who make wrong assumptions about administrators because of past events and experiences. The following may make this easier to understand.

THEY ARE ALL THAT WAY

Over the years as I have participated in medical staff meetings, I've often heard physicians say that we cannot trust the administration because of some event which occurred sometimes as much as 20 years in the past. It may even have involved an administrator no longer at the hospital. However, the event caused the physician not to trust any administration and laid the groundwork for the Great Divide. At the same time, I have been in administrative meetings and heard exactly the same thing said about a physician who in the past had misrepresented or failed to follow through with a project. This long-past event colored the administration's mistrust and carried it forward. Amazingly, both sides would base their persistent judgments on events occurring many years earlier, often involving people who were no longer working there.. Ironically, both sides made the same incorrect assumptions. This failure to move past the previous events shows a marked misunderstanding of how people change with circumstances and time. Institutional memory is very important, but it can be a hindrance if it is used to interpret new events based on long past history.

INCLUDE THE PHYSICIANS EARLY

Another tendency I have observed is one in which administrators start a new program that will affect the physicians' workplace (the hospital), and yet they fail to include the medical staff in the project's early planning discussions. Sometimes this can be as simple as a change in the food service at the hospital, which the physicians only learn about when patients start complaining to them as they make rounds, or it can be as complex as building a complicated new surgical suite. Physicians work every day in the hospital setting, and it is important they feel some ownership of their work environment. When hospital administration plans an initiative, starts to train the staff, and starts the process without getting the buy-in of the medical staff, it can lead to the failure of the project and further widen the divide between physicians and administrators. Waiting to invite the physicians to buy in late in the process leads to a loss of ownership. Physicians feel they have been left out of the planning and implementation of the new initiative, and see this as a sign that the administration does not value their input.

Many times the administration has made some attempt at outreach but has not effectively communicated the initiative with the physicians. This seems like a simple idea: *include the physicians who practice in the facility in any major changes, which will affect them.* Remember, the medical staff is made up of many bright and talented people and should be seen by the administration as a great source of good ideas. However, many administrators have made the same error over and over again by not including the physicians in the early stages of the development of a new project.

The Squeaky Wheel Gets the Grease

The process of purchasing new equipment and supplies for a hospital can be very complicated and expensive. Done effectively, it involves people at many levels of the organization and is conducted in a way that is financially sound for the healthcare institution. In the past, when purchasing new equipment, many institutions tended to listen only to the physicians who were the loudest complainers. This often led to the purchase of equipment, which was not really needed or was suited only for use on a small number of patients, and it was not always economical for the institution.

In order to avoid this problem, many institutions now include multiple physicians in the equipment purchasing process. Physicians can help a hospital make informed decisions about purchasing medical equipment. This inclusion has increased physicians' understanding of the economics driving the hospital and healthcare in general. It has also given hospitals a better idea of the real needs of the medical staff members and their patients.

Closing the Communication Gap

As we have discussed, medical staff members and hospital administrators have often gone their separate ways when trying to address patient needs. Because of the need for alignment to address the hospital's financial issues as well as the best practice of care for their patients, both administrators and physicians must learn to communicate effectively and successfully. There are many new and inventive ways this is being addressed across the country. We will discuss this further in future chapters. In the meantime, here are some of the basics of building a culture of communication.

Rules of Engagement
For administration:
- Listen to your physicians
- Involve your physicians early in the process
- Communicate in multiple ways
- Set up liaisons to visit physicians on a regular basis
- Round on your physicians
- Set up physician feedback groups to meet regularly with administration
- Include outlying physicians in your feedback group
- Get feedback continuously from your medical staff
- Train your physicians in business practices
- Respond to physician concerns in a timely fashion

Doctor Time and Hospital Time
Finally, one of the biggest errors I have observed in my years working with both physicians and administrators is a disparity in time and response. For many years, I have observed 'physician time' as occurring in 24 hours. As physicians, we are trained to respond to a patient's need as quickly as possible. We are given a problem and we solve it. That is how we are trained, and that is how we expect others to behave.

This, of course, collides with the world of administration. The necessary bureaucracy of a hospital does not allow for, nor can it respond with, quick answers. When a hospital has to make a major change, it takes time. So physicians work in an expected turnaround time of 24 hours, while hospital turnaround time can be as much as a year.

Many times, the real mistake is the failure to follow up and the failure to keep physicians informed about the process. In best practices, we see health systems address the concerns of physicians in a timely manner and respond with continuous updates as the process moves forward. This helps physicians understand how the process works and the complications that occur because of the needs of a health system. By keeping physicians apprised of the progress, the system encourages a sense of value for concerns.

Often the hospital's response is not the answer a physician wants to hear, but physicians appreciate the fact that the hospital has taken their concern seriously and given them a reasonable answer about why the process could not move forward.

This is one of the early lessons physicians learn when they begin working in administrative medicine: *the hospital is a large and complicated environment, and a quick fix may cause more problems than it corrects.* Because physicians want to fix the problem, they do not always appreciate or understand the bureaucracy and how fixing one problem can lead to problems for other parts of the system. This is especially true for new physician administrators.

* * * * *

As we move forward, we must work to bring physicians and administrators into the same world. Healthcare is a team sport, and to do the best for our patients we must work together and understand each other's needs and how best to reach the common goal of great patient care.

Chapter 7 – Whoa, Too Much Information

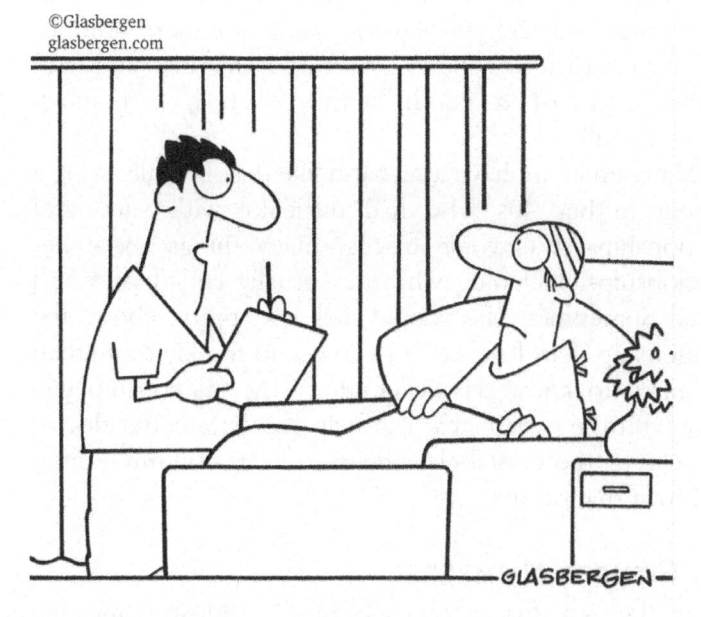

"You caught a virus from your computer and we had to erase your brain. I hope you've got a back-up copy!"

IN THIS CHAPTER, we will look at the problems and concerns of our digital world and how our multiple ways of communicating are leading us to data overload. We are seeing a lot of noise and very little true communication. We truly do have a situation with 'too much information' in the form of data making the true picture of patients' needs fuzzy and clouded.

* * * * *

For 28 years I was privileged to care for patients as a family physician. During this time of caring for patients, I learned a great deal about them and their lives. Sometimes I learned more than I really needed or wanted to know. Sometimes you feel you have *too much information*. One of my favorite cartoons shows a doctor waving his hands and backing out of a room, saying "Whoa, too much information!"

Many times we have a scenario like this. I recall seeing a patient in her 40s who had difficulty with successful relationships. We would discuss many things about her relationships, including why they usually ended on a sad note. Sometimes she would tell me more about the relationship than I needed to know, and frankly more than I wanted to know. However, that's the relationship you have with the patient that can help you be a better doctor because of the crystal-clear heart-to-heart communication and trust that occurs.

My Fitness Numbers

Over the last few years, the fitness industry and the computer industry have both made many advances to help patients keep track of their daily exercise goals. This can serve as a great motivator for people to exercise more.

The invention of personal devices that keep up with each step you take during the day and record your heart rate, pulse, blood pressure, and even in some instances the amount of calories consumed are now readily available for everyone. One of the many innovative designs includes the ability to download a patient's exercise activities to their medical record. The data, of course, is important for a physician to know. Good feedback on regular exercise and dietary habits can be beneficial. However, the amount of information and data coming from these devices can overwhelm the electronic medical record the physician has in their office. It also presents a problem for the physician who is now required to know the data because it is in the medical record as a record of the activities of the patient. The data takes up space on the record and of course takes time and effort on the part of the physician who is now expected to review all of the data being downloaded to the medical record. Can you imagine the amount of data produced by 200 of your patients downloading their monthly activity? So we have a dilemma: how do we best get the information the patient and physician need to share without overwhelming the system with data which is either unimportant or will not make a difference in how the physician cares for the patient? Thus we have the challenge of *too much data.*

THE EMR (THE PRODUCTIVITY KILLER)

As we have discussed in previous chapters, the introduction of the electronic medical record (EMR) has been both a blessing and a curse for physicians. It has required significant changes in the day-to-day interactions of physicians with their patients and with other physicians. In some instances, it has improved communication, and in other instances, it has limited communication and made it much harder. There are examples of problems with records generated in the hospital, the emergency room, the doctor's office, and other areas of medical care. Let's look at a few cases of how the EMR has generated problems that can lead to medical errors and patient injury.

The emergency room is a place where the sickest and the most acutely ill are treated. Working there requires quick thinking and accurate responses on the part of the staff. Time is of the essence. In order to provide the best patient care, a record of the visit must be generated. Because of the liability risk, the record must be very accurate and complete.

With the introduction of EMRs, we have introduced new obstacles to good care. When a patient goes to the emergency room, their medical record must accurately reflect the care given. Unfortunately, many of the electronic medical record companies and software developers have not clearly understood the workflow of the emergency department physician and staff. As a result, the software does not simulate the real workflow that happens when a patient is seen in the emergency room. Because of these disparities, the patient medical record generated in the emergency room often does not clearly represent what was done or the problems the patient presented with during the visit. Let's look at the following example.

Mrs. Martin is a 42-year-old female patient followed by her family doctor, Dr. Bill Williams. One Saturday afternoon, Mrs. Martin developed symptoms of chest tightness, weakness, and diaphoresis (profuse sweating). Mrs. Martin goes to the emergency room, where Dr. Phillips sees her. The medical record is generated through the electronic health record used by the hospital in the emergency department.

Unfortunately, the electronic medical record used in the emergency room is a different type than the one used by the hospitalist department that cares for patients admitted to the hospital. To add to the confusion, the electronic medical record Mrs. Martin's family physician uses in his office is also a different type. The groundwork for poor communication is already laid because of the reality that none of the three EMRs directly communicate with each other.

After Mrs. Martin is seen and evaluated in the emergency room, it is determined that her chest pain may or may not be cardiac in origin. Due to risk factors of smoking and a family history of heart disease, Mrs. Martin is admitted to the hospitalist service for overnight observation and a nuclear exercise treadmill test the next morning. She has an uneventful hospitalization, but that is not the case for the hospitalist taking care of Mrs. Martin.

Because the emergency room electronic medical record does not 'talk' directly to the hospital electronic medical record, very important information has to be transferred from one system to the other either by hospital staff or an electronic bridge between systems. This allows another interaction where information relevant to Mrs. Martin's condition and care might not be completely communicated when the records are transferred.

In this case, Mrs. Martin is given medication to which she is allergic, and she has an allergic reaction. Fortunately, it was a minimal reaction, but it could have been completely avoided had the two systems been able to communicate effectively with each other.

The hospitalist views Mrs. Martin's exercise test in the morning and determines she does not have cardiac disease. Mrs. Martin is discharged and another medical record is completed for her visit. One week later, Mrs. Martin goes to see her family physician, Dr. Williams, for a follow-up post-discharge review. Dr. Williams is happy to see Mrs. Martin, but there is a problem. Because his office's electronic medical record and the electronic medical record from the hospital, along with the emergency room records, do not interact with Dr. Williams' system, he does not have a record of Mrs. Martin's hospitalization. This means Dr. Williams has to ask his staff to obtain the records from the hospital, further delaying his ability to care for Mrs. Martin. Dr. Williams has another difficulty: the amount of data received from the hospital, and particularly the emergency room record. During her initial evaluation, Mrs. Martin was in the emergency room for two hours and 15 minutes. However, 22 pages of information were generated from the emergency room visit. Somewhere in the emergency room documents is important information for Dr. Williams. However, Dr. Williams does not have the time to look through the voluminous medical record to find what he needs to know to properly care for Mrs. Martin.

Compounding this problem, the medication reconciliation done in the emergency room and the hospitalist record of the medication do not match. This may have contributed to Mrs. Martin's allergic reaction in the hospital. As in the emergency room record, the hospitalist record has an overwhelming amount of information generated, so it is hard for Dr. Williams to extract pertinent laboratory data and care information from Mrs. Martin's hospitalization. Dr. Williams needs to know exactly what occurred, and what he needs to do going forward to care for his patient.

This is an example of too much information being produced and delivered in a way that overwhelms the recipient. The volume of data produced is far more than the doctor who cares for Mrs. Martin in the outpatient world can process quickly in order to make decisions about her care going forward.

The incompatibility of different electronic medical record systems also leads to confusion and patient harm. We now have in excess of 400 different electronic medical record software packages available for physician outpatient practices. Unfortunately, many of them are incompatible with each other, so the ability to convey information in a clear and concise way is lost. This was a major error on the part of regulators, who did not make intercommunication a prime requirement of the development of electronic medical records. Multiple operating systems increase the likelihood of poor communication and patient harm.

Although they may be expert developers, software development by non-physicians has increased the volume of information generated that does not directly improve patient care. This is apparent in Mrs. Martin's 22-page emergency room record. The sheer volume of information contained in her records is extremely risky for Mrs. Martin. Important information about what really occurred in the hospital and what Dr. Williams needs to know is lost in the records from the emergency room and the separate hospitalist records. What's needed? A concise, connected record in order to help Dr. Williams work with the other physicians to give seamless care to Mrs. Martin and keep her well.

Lost in Translation

In the early 1990's our family medicine group took a great leap of faith and became a beta test site for one of the early electronic medical records systems. Being a beta site means you are an early user, and you get to find out what works and what doesn't. We were excited about the possibilities for our patients and for the practice of medicine. Because of the many promises of better care promoted by the electronic medical record developer, we saw a great opportunity to improve care. We were told the electronic medical record would allow us to share our records directly with other physicians, and not only would they see our records, but we would see their records of our patients' visits with them. We learned the software would detect drug interactions, promoting a safer patient experience. Electronic medical records would allow us to search our data for pertinent information, watching for changes and trends to help improve care. It would only take a few simple commands to accomplish these things. The promise of intercommunication between systems would help the specialist and the family physician share information that would streamline patient care for both physicians.

Fast-forward a few years: instead of system compatibility, we often have an inability to share the full medical record, and in some instances, an inability to share any of the patients' records. Who does this affect? Primary care doctors referring patients to subspecialists. It affects the emergency room physician who cannot see the record of a patient's visit to a different emergency room in the same community one week earlier. Sometimes the primary care physician employed by the hospital is unable to share his or her office records with the hospitalist because of the lack of compatibility between the two EMR systems which are on two different platforms and do not directly share information. The promise of cross-communication, the ability for physicians to share the patient's complete record, is a wonderful yet elusive goal we have not met. It continues to undermine the promised benefits of the electronic medical record and cause poor communication.

As health care providers, it's up to us to help software developers achieve the goal of sharing necessary patient information seamlessly. This in turn moves us toward higher standards of outstanding patient care.

THE PLATFORM IS ONLY AS GOOD AS ITS CONTENT

The ultimate goal of ready access to electronic medical records is to help us as physicians better care for our patients. This means that we need to actively participate with software developers to refine and strengthen their platforms. The electronic medical record is only as good as the information placed in it. For example, it is important that medication reconciliation be accomplished quickly and accurately so all physicians and staff are aware of the actual medications a patient is taking. Sharing pharmacy records and collecting an accurate list is essential to patient safety. The same is true of an accurate allergy list and past medical history. This basic patient care information must be entered into the medical record immediately in order to protect the patient's safety.

CAN'T SEE THE FOREST FOR THE TREES

Other possible risks to patient safety include selecting medications from a drop-down menu in the electronic medical record. While this can make it easier to prescribe a medication, it can also pose a health risk if the menu is not easily readable to the ordering physician. Mistakes in prescribing and ordering drugs can cause harm to the patient, as can drug interactions and allergic reactions. As we saw in the case of Mrs. Martin, failing to have an accurate allergy record can also lead to a patient receiving medications to which they are allergic. The automatic generation of long, confusing emergency room records can make it impossible to see the forest for the trees.

CUTTING AND PASTING

Another major concern is the use of cut and paste techniques in daily hospital records. Copying and pasting information is a way to easily populate a note. However, it can generate information that is not helpful and does not give a clear picture of the care of the patient nor the state of the patient's medical condition at the time the record was produced. Inaccurate records can cause patient harm and possibly lead to medical liability and legal issues. Cutting and pasting information can also generate possible false claims, which can be interpreted as Medicare fraud.

THE IMPORTANCE OF CLEAR RECORDS

As physicians, we have an obligation to develop a clear, concise patient medical record that helps other caregivers understand the patient's medical care. So far the electronic medical records currently available miss the mark of simplification and interoperability. The amount of time needed to document, update, maintain, and access electronic medical records continues to limit physician productivity.

In fact, according to a landmark study in Mayo Clinic Proceedings[1], the demands of electronic record keeping also contribute heavily to "physician burnout," which more than half of doctors experience. One of the underlying issues is that most EMRs in the US today were originally designed to be utilized for billing purposes rather than to enhance clinical care or the coordination of care.[2]

PHYSICIAN PUSH BACK

Recently the AMA and the Rand Corporation surveyed physicians on what they felt were the biggest challenges facing the practice of medicine today.[3]

The following are some of the findings from the AMA/RAND study.

"We found that factors in several broad categories were important determinants of physician and processional satisfaction, as detailed below. In our judgment, the most novel and important findings concerned *how physician's perceptions of quality of care and use of electronic health record affected professional satisfaction.* The findings for quality and electronic health records were:

1. *Electronic health records.* EHRs have important effects on physician professional satisfaction, both positive and negative. In the practices we studied, physicians approved of EHRs in concept, describing better ability to remotely access patient information and improvements in quality of care. Physicians, practice leaders, and other staff also noted the potential of EHRs to further improve both patient care and professional satisfaction in the future, as EHR technology, especially user interfaces and health information exchanges, improves.

However, for many physicians, the current state of the EHR technology significantly worsened professional satisfaction in multiple ways. Poor EHR usability, time-consuming data entry, interference with face-to-face patient care, inefficient and less fulfilling work content, inability to exchange health information between the EHR products, and degradation of clinical documentation were prominent sources of professional dissatisfaction. Some of these problems were more prominent among senior physicians and those lacking scribes, transcriptionists, and other staff to support data entry or manage information flow. Physicians across the full range of specialties and practice models described other problems, including but not limited to frustrations with receiving template-generated notes (i.e. degradation of clinical documentation). In addition, EHRs have been more expensive than anticipated for some practices, threatening practice financial sustainability.

Some practices reported taking steps to address the cause of physician dissatisfaction with EHRs. Most commonly, the steps allowed multiple modes of data entry and employment of other staff members in order to help physicians focus their interaction with EHRs on activities truly requiring the physicians training.

2. *Collegiality, fairness, and respect.* Physicians' perceptions of collegiality, fairness, and respect were key determinants of professional satisfaction. Physicians reported four main areas in which these constructs operated: relationships with colleagues in the practice, relationships with providers outside the practice, relationships with patients, and relationships with payers.

Within the practice, frequent meetings with other physicians and allied health professionals foster greater collegiality. Physicians who no longer co-own practices observe that when personal familiarity with their former partners decreases, it leads to lower overall morale.

Physicians reported limited but important specialty specific frustrations with unfairness and disrespect when interacting with other providers. For surgeons, these concerns surface most prominently in writing hospital call duties. For primary care physicians, interaction with other physicians was problematic when primary care physicians were treated as subservient."[4]

The AMA/RAND report goes on to say that better EHR usability should be an industry-wide priority and a precondition for EHR certification. Speeding improvement of EHR usability may require direct incentives for EHR vendors. Until EHR usability improves dramatically, to the point that direct interacting with the EHR neither creates additional, excessive clerical work for physicians nor distracts from patient care, removing regulatory and legal barriers to using other practice staff to interact directly with EHRs will allow physicians more time to perform work that requires physician training.

* * * * *

As we move forward with the use of electronic medical records, physicians need to play a more active role in helping develop a clear, user-friendly electronic medical record. The government cannot continue to add regulatory burdens such as Meaningful Use Three (all of the requirements that physicians must meet to receive their incentives and avoid any penalties) and still expect to reach the goal of interoperability.[2] At this point, the promise of the electronic medical record to help physicians provide consistent high-quality care for their patients is still a distant goal.

Chapter 8 – The Death of Professionalism

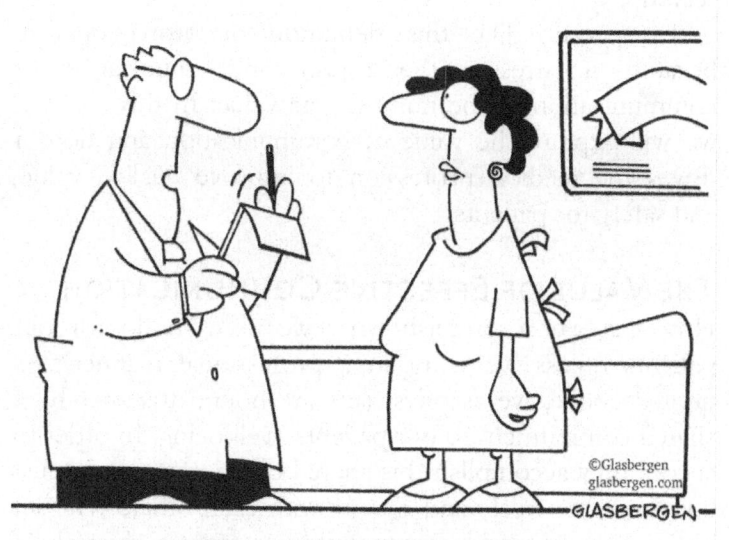

"I'm prescribing a squiggly line, two slanted loops, and something that looks like a P or J."

PROFESSIONALISM. IT UNDERSCORES not only what we do, but how, and why. In this chapter we'll examine missed opportunities and their consequences, and take a look at the lessons of legibility.

* * * * *

In their 2002 paper presented in the Journal of the American Medical Association, R. M. Epstein and E. M. Hundert defined professionalism this way:

"Professional competence is the habitual and judicious use of communication, knowledge, technical skills, clinical reasoning, emotions, values, and reflection in daily practice for the benefit of the individual and community being served."[1]

I especially like this definition of professionalism because it stresses the power and importance of communication as the number one value. In this chapter, we will explore the value of communication and how it drives the medical profession to improve quality, value, and safety for patients.

THE VALUE OF EFFECTIVE COMMUNICATION

How can we accomplish what we need to do for our patients unless we work in a professional manner? As quoted above, we as physicians are bound together by a shared commitment to our patients' well-being. In order to successfully accomplish this shared commitment, we must communicate freely and openly with each other. Without physician-to-physician communication, we run the risk of harming our patients. Physician handoffs, referrals, and even the simple task of ordering a chest x-ray all require proper communication.

The following is an example of how a failure to communicate can be dangerous to a patient:

It is 2:30 in the morning and a trauma has occurred. The EMS crew brings a 35-year-old male patient to the emergency room. The patient has been involved in a head-on collision in which another person died. The patient is unconscious and no family members are present to give a history. The emergency room physician evaluates the patient and orders a trauma CT scan. The radiologist reviews the scan, having only the history that the patient was in a MVA (motor vehicle accident). The radiologist must review several hundred CT slices and determine if there are any underlying surgical or medical conditions on them. This situation occurs every day in emergency rooms across the country.

The events described above may seem straightforward, but they can have horrible consequences for a patient. In just this single event, we see three separate times where the patient was handed off and the opportunity to communicate a thorough patient history was lost. The patient is unconscious, and cannot give any history of the events. The patient also cannot give any history of his underlying medical condition.

MISSED OPPORTUNITY #1

The EMS crew saw and understood how the accident occurred. They can give a history of the type of force used to cause the patient's injuries and they have the history of the patient's symptoms and vital signs obtained at the scene of the accident and during the ambulance ride to the hospital. This communication is vitally important to the patient's safety and care. If this history is relayed accurately to the emergency room physician, the patient's care will be more directed.

MISSED OPPORTUNITY #2

The next handoff occurs when the emergency room physician orders the trauma CT scan. If the emergency room physician does not give a history to the radiologist of exactly what they are concerned about based on their examination of the patient in the emergency room, then the physician has not done their job. In order to be sure no injury is missed, a thorough history of the motor vehicle accident and the force of the trauma can make a big difference in what the radiologist is able to discern when looking at the CT scan.

MISSED OPPORTUNITY #3

The third handoff occurs when the CT scan report is sent back to the emergency room physician. If there was evidence of an injury, which was not clearly specified, then the emergency room physician could not complete their job.

Events like these, all seemingly minor on their own, can lead to death and/or long-term disability for the patient. We cannot stress just how important good communication is when a patient's care is transferred and a handoff is completed.

A LIFE-CHANGING CONSEQUENCE

In this case, because the radiologist did not know about the head-on collision, he failed to see a small bleed on the patient's scan which became a severe bleed and led to the patient suffering permanent brain damage. This might have been avoided had a good hand-off occurred.

As Harvard Law Professor Einer Elhauge points out in his book *The Fragmentation of U.S. Health Care: Causes and Solutions*, it's often the patient that is responsible for coordinating the efforts of the various doctors — a task which is not only time-consuming and costly, but also requires professional experience.

Without a proper system in place to improve communication between the growing number of people involved in a patient's care, it can be difficult to tell just who is responsible for following up when things fall through the cracks.[2]

HISTORY MAKES A DIFFERENCE

Every day in this country, millions of x-rays and scans are ordered on patients to address their medical condition. Many times, very little appropriate history is sent with the order for the x-ray. When the radiologist reviews the films, they are at a disadvantage, as they do not know what concerns the ordering physician has and what they are looking for. Radiologists can and do respond appropriately when they have the history to guide them as they interpret the films.

THE LIMITATIONS OF CONVENIENCE

Many of the new electronic medical records have pull-down menus for history completion when ordering a radiological test. Often these menus are limited and the history is not accurate or detailed enough to help the radiologist interpret the films. Again, if there is important information to communicate, this can be done best by talking directly to the radiologist or leaving a handwritten note or dictation in the record when ordering the exam. This important detail can and often does lead to patient harm when not done correctly.

A MATTER OF LEGIBILITY

Prior to the advent of the electronic medical record, the running joke was, "physicians have terrible hand writing."

102 | PHYSICIANS SHOULD TALK

The writing was so bad that many times nurses literally would have to guess what the physician really meant when they received a handwritten order. The following examples show just how bad physician written orders can be, and point out the real risk of the wrong medicine being ordered on the wrong patient at the wrong time.

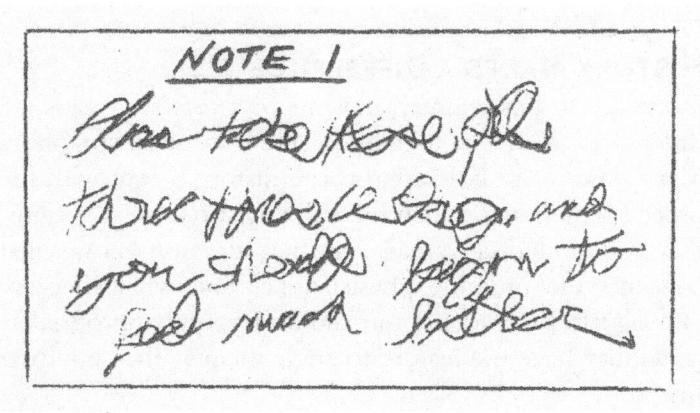

Figure 4.[3]

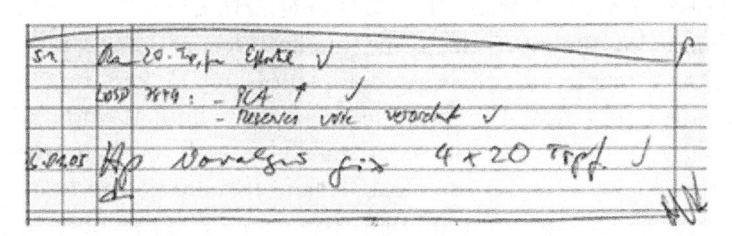

Figure 5.[4]

With the advent of the electronic medical record, physicians can type their orders into a computer, making the order legible. However, with the reliance on limited menus and drop-down options, many times the wrong option is chosen, leading to a new kind of medical error. This is why good communication can have a significant effect on the quality of patient care and safety.

HIPAA AND COMMUNICATION

In 1996 the U.S. government introduced the Health Insurance Portability and Accountability Act. HIPAA, as it is now commonly known, was put into law to help manage patient information and protect the privacy and confidentiality of that information. It preceded the adoption of the electronic medical record and was passed to help protect patients and their right to personal privacy. Under this act, patients have a right to ask that information be withheld. However, if that request is not made, patients' information may be released under the appropriate conditions.[5]

HIPAA has caused significant concerns because of the high fines that can be levied against physicians, hospitals, and their staffs for non-compliance. Initially the rules were misunderstood and as so often happen, many barriers were put in place, which made it harder for appropriate and necessary patient information to be moved and shared. The law was meant to cover EHR records, but now encompasses all forms of communication, thus adding cost and complexity to the sharing of medical information during treatment. As time has gone on, the rules are better understood and appropriate safeguards have been put in place through compliance plans and patient data monitoring. However, this understanding has come at a cost. Because so much patient information is stored online, there continues to be a great risk of a data breach and the loss of patient information. As discussed earlier, many hospitals have had breaches resulting in significant fines.

Good communication can still occur. In light of HIPAA, when discussing patient information, we adhere to the following guidelines:

1. First – be sure that others who have no need to know about the patient's information cannot overhear your conversation.
2. Second – be sure the information is being relayed to another individual who is directly involved in the care of the patient.
3. Third – be sure the information being communicated is necessary for the care of the patient.

Some recent examples of HIPAA violations primarily involve data breaches and lost devices:

1. The Utah Department of Health confirmed that a server containing personal health information of some 780,000 patients was intentionally hacked.
2. Emory Healthcare reported misplacing 10 backup discs, which contained information for more than 315,000 patients. It also contained Social Security numbers, patient names, surgery dates, diagnoses, and procedure codes.
3. South Carolina Department of Health and Human Services reported a data breach, which started in January 2012 when an employee compiled data on more than 228,000 people and transmitted the data to a private email account.
4. Alere, a Livermore, California-based company which provides home health anticoagulation monitoring services, reported an unencrypted laptop containing patient names, social security numbers, addresses, and diagnoses was stolen from an employee's car.
5. Florida's Memorial Health System notified

some 102,000 patients about a breach that occurred in 2012. The affected patients were told that an employee working for an affiliated physician's office improperly accessed patient names, dates of birth, and social security numbers.[6]

* * * * *

All of these violations resulted in employees losing their jobs and heavy fines for not appropriately safeguarding patient information. Something as simple as a conversation in an elevator overheard by a third party can lead to the loss of patient information and the invasion of patient privacy. So as we move forward and work together to communicate more effectively, we must always keep in mind the risk of a HIPAA violation and the ongoing need for patient privacy.

Chapter 9 – Everything Old is New Again

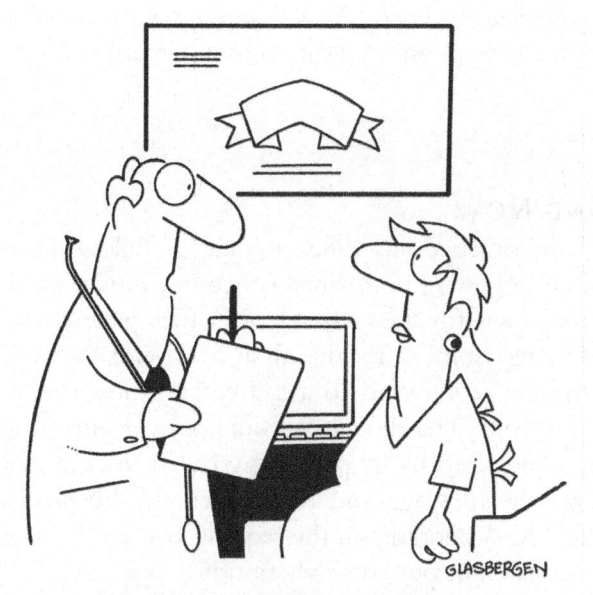

"Laughter is the best medicine, but there's a $50 co-pay."

WHILE MOST OF us were dragged kicking and screaming into electronic medical records, most physicians would not want to return to those earlier days of paper and pen. However, today's electronic medical records can seem like the Tower of Babel as we have over 460 different electronic medical record systems, very few of which actually share information with other systems. As healthcare and especially the practice of medicine moves at a faster pace and our ever-expanding knowledge base continues to grow, instead of longing for the old days, we can make smarter use of our tools for communicating. By so doing, we will help our patients receive higher quality, safer care.

Let's begin this chapter by sharing my personal experience in how communication has changed over my 32 years of medical practice. We'll wrap up with a list of guidelines for better communication useful in any setting.

* * * * *

Then and Now

I began my practice in 1982, joining a fellow family physician and opening up a small office in Florida. At the time we took calls for the hospital, our office patients, and several nursing homes. In the first few years we used beepers (pagers) connected to a call center known as the doctor's directory. The directory would answer our phone after hours and beep us by pager. We called the directory back to get the message and then called the hospital or patient directly, depending on the request. Invariably, when we were on call and out somewhere not near a telephone, we would get a call requiring us to find a pay phone, which in most places today no longer exist.

Over time, we learned where all the local pay phones were in order to answer calls as quickly as possible.

Not long after that, we graduated to using two-way radios over which the directory would contact us and connect us to the nurse or patient who was calling. Unfortunately, when we pressed the button to talk, we would cut out the other end of the line, so many times the conversation consisted of both sides talking over each other with very little information being transmitted. However, the good news was we no longer had to find a pay phone.

Following the use of the two-way radio, we next received our first cellular phone, which was a bag phone. It was 18" x 18" and contained a large battery along with the telephone. These allowed us to return pages from a car or wherever we might be. This, of course, made calls much easier. However, the phone was bulky and the battery short-lived.

Next came smaller versions of the cell phone. This was considered a major breakthrough in communications. The original cell phones were basic telephones, but they were good for calling back and returning patient calls. Later, we added the ability to read emails and text messages and respond to a call without having to talk with anyone.

Now, we basically carry a computer in our pocket that allows us to send, receive, and respond to emails, texts, and voice communications.

Ironically, while we have made great progress in having multiple ways to communicate, we have in fact gone backwards. We now send lots of information, but many times the clutter overwhelms us and we fail to get the right message to the right person at the right time.

Who Needs to Talk?

As we have discussed in previous chapters, we depend on clear, concise ways to communicate so we can improve the quality of patient care and safety. When we communicate in a timely, understandable way, good information is sent and received, leading to better patient outcomes. Let's look at an episode of patient care and see the many ways communication occurs and how it can affect patient outcomes.

Our patient, Mrs. Larson, is a 45-year-old female patient of Dr. Harris who comes to his office with a chief complaint of shortness of breath. First she comes to the lobby, where the front office staff greets her and determines how quickly she needs to see the doctor. This is the first face-to-face communication event between the patient and the office receptionist. The receptionist then discusses the case with Dr. Harris's nurse, who brings Mrs. Larson back to the exam room and alerts Dr. Harris of the situation. Dr. Harris interacts with the patient and she communicates her history of shortness of breath. After the patient evaluation, Dr. Harris determines she should be admitted to the local hospital for further testing. Dr. Harris' nurse calls the admissions office and explains the need for the patient admission and then Mrs. Larson is accepted to the hospital for admission.

The next round of communication occurs when Mrs. Larson sees the hospitalist at the hospital and again relates her history of shortness of breath. She is also seen by the floor nurses and encounters laboratory and radiologic personnel, who interact with Mrs. Larson as well as with the floor nurses. The hospitalist then consults a pulmonologist for further evaluation.

After several days in the hospital, Mrs. Larson is better and is discharged home. Prior to leaving, she sees the discharge planner, and appointments are made for a follow-up visit with her family physician, Dr. Harris, and a pulmonologist. Records are dictated by the hospitalist and the pulmonologist and are sent to Dr. Harris for his follow-up appointment with Mrs. Larson.

In an ideal world, the patient would be seen within five days of discharge, and at the time of the visit, the records from the hospital would be available to Dr. Harris. However, what occurs many times is more like this: Mrs. Larson comes to Dr. Harris's office after her discharge and is finally seen three weeks later, and still the discharge summary and hospital records are not in Dr. Harris's office. Neither Dr. Harris nor the patient really knows what care was given in the hospital. At a minimum, there is a delay in care while both records are retrieved from the hospital, or worse, the patient goes back to the hospital before her follow-up appointment and is readmitted.

Let's review the many times there were opportunities for communication failures while Mrs. Larson was treated during her brief hospitalization. Three physicians were directly involved in her care. Several other physicians were indirectly involved in interpreting test results for Mrs. Larson. Hospital staff, nurses, and other personnel were also involved in caring for Mrs. Larson during her hospitalization. You can clearly see how many times poor communication can affect the patient's health and wellbeing.

How to Communicate, Let me Count the Ways

Today the options for transmitting information continue to expand. We can use emails or send text messages. We have multiple software programs including Vocera, Snapchat, Spok, Volte, Perfect Serve, and the What's App, all of which are designed to help facilitate rapid, accurate communication about patient care issues. These programs work through the Internet to send HIPPA-protected information to the physician, facilitating timely patient care. They allow physicians to get real-time information and make decisions about care without having to be at the bedside reading the chart. As length of hospital stay has become more important and the need for quick reporting of lab test results has increased, these software programs help improve patient care and successful treatment outcomes.

While there are some risks for security of the information and for data over-saturation, which always have to be considered, these can be a great addition to the physician's essential tool kit for good patient care.

HIPAA

In 2003, the federal government passed the Health Insurance Portability Accountability Act designed to facilitate use of electronic medical record systems with the main goal of transferring information about patients among health care workers involved in the patient's care. Patient-protected information, or PHI, is shared many times, and with the advent of new technologies, the ability to share that information continues to evolve. HIPAA-compliant technologies are an invaluable tool for healthcare providers and physicians who must communicate among themselves in order to give the best care possible. As we adopt more and better communication technologies, the basic security of that information must be paramount at all times. This is a challenge we will continue to face in light of the difficulty of protecting patient information. Violation of the act can lead to significant financial penalties. As we have discussed in earlier chapters, the main point to remember is that in any of your choices for software or communication technologies, always make sure they are HIPAA compliant.

How Can I Find What I Need to know?

With the explosion of new technologies and ready access via computer to more data, we now face a new dilemma: too much information and the difficulty to determine what data is most important for patient care. Health care outcomes can and will be improved with the use of new technologies, but we must be able to wade through all of the information and see what really needs to be addressed in order to take the best care of our patients.

The following is a medical record produced by an emergency room visit. The record has been changed to protect the PHI. The information is presented to show how difficult it is to address all of the needed data sets which the insurance company, the federal government and the health organization requires and still produce a record which is usable for the care of the individual patient. See if you can tell what information the primary care physician needs in order to continue caring for the patient who was seen and treated in the emergency room.

EMERGENCY RECORD

NURSING PROCEDURE: NURSE NOTES (2) 40-CED
NURSES NOTES: Patient examined by physician. Notes

NURSING ASSESSMENT: ENT (21.35 CED
CONSTITUTIONAL PED: Complex assessment performed, Patient arrives ambulatory, accompanied by parent. History obtained from parent, Patient alert, **Patient, ill appearing**, Patient interactive and playful, Patient consolable, Patient appropriately dressed, Skin warm, and dry, and normal in color, Capillary refill less than 2 seconds, Mucous membranes pink, and moist.
PAIN: **on a scale 0-10 patient rates pain as 4**.
ENT: **Discharge, thin**, Mucous membranes pink, and moist, Able to swallow, Speech normal, no associated fever, Notes: pt **and mother state he started c/o throat pain today and has had a runny nose for 4-5 days, pt denies any other pain**.
RESPIRATORY/CHEST: Respiratory assessment findings include respiratory effort easy, Respirations regular, Conversing normally, no signs of distress, Breath sounds clear, Neck and chest exam findings include trachea midline, Chest expansion equal, Chest movement symmetrical, no associated cough noted, no associated fever.

MEDICATION SERVICE (21.48 JQ)
prednisoLONE: Order: prednisoLONE (prednisolone) – **Dose:** 35 mg : Oral
   Schedule: STAT
   Ordered by
   Entered by ▓▓▓▓▓▓▓▓▓▓ Thu Sep 01, 2016 21:45 ,
   Co-signed by ▓▓▓▓▓▓▓▓▓▓ Thu Sep 01, 2016 21:45.
   Acknowledged by ▓▓▓▓▓▓▓▓▓▓ Thu Sep 01, 2016 21:46
   Documented as given by ▓▓▓▓▓▓▓▓▓▓ Thu Sep 01, 2016 21:48
Patient, Medication, Dose, Route and Time verified prior to administration.
Amount given: 35 mg. Site: Medication administered P.O., Correct patient, time, route, dose and medication confirmed prior to administration, Patient advised of actions and side-effects prior to administration, Allergies confirmed and medications reviewed prior to administration, Patient in position of comfort, Side rails up, Cart in lowest position, Family at bedside, Call light in reach.

ALLERGY (19.37)
NO KNOWN ALLERGIES by Interface.
NO KNOWN DRUG ALLERGIES by Interface.
NO KNOWN FOOD ALLERGIES by Interface.

ADMIN
PATIENT DATA CHANGE: Race: (none), KG Weight: 17.6. (19 37 AWH)
   A08 581DEF1B-68DF-4A11-B2E1-CA18021E944E by Interface, Name: (19.37)
   A08 138472113 by Interface, Ethnicity: (none). (19.37)
   A08 B601C1AB-D558-4CD6-A24F-8CE7E962EC55 by Interface. (19.37)
   A08 138472114 by Interface, Ethnicity: (none). (19.37)
   A08 3211BA34-211B-4CEC-97FC-53AFF474CFB1 by Interface. (19 37)
   A08 138472139 by Interface. (19.38)

Prepared: Sat Sep 03, 2016 12:08 by Interface Page: 4 of 5
SEE CHART IN ED PULSECHECK APPLICATION ARCHIVE FOR CHART ENTRY DATES AND TIMES.

Figure 6.[1]

Can you determine what the physician should do? This record is the perfect example of too much data and too many requirements by payers and the government. Unfortunately the information the physician needs to take best care of the patient is not readily apparent in this record, and many times it's not even in the record because the record was designed to address the needs of the payer and the computer software developer, not the end user and the workflows that must occur in the practice of medicine. Please review the next record, giving particular attention to the synopsis that is really the essence of what the physician needs to know about the visit to the emergency room. The synopsis summarizes the event, giving the doctor essential information about what was done and what still needed to be done. As we continue to improve the electronic medical record, we must get to a simplified, easily understandable record that can be used efficiently by physicians to care for their patients.

EMERGENCY RECORD

IV therapy indicated for medication administration, IV established, to the right hand, using a 20 gauge catheter, in one attempt.
SAFETY: Side rails up, Cart/Stretcher in lowest position, Family at bedside, Call light within reach, Hospital ID band on.

NURSING PROCEDURE: NURSE NOTES
NURSES NOTES: Notes: CRMC faxed medical release form for any recent labs or CT/MRI that were performed.
Notes: dr clemmons notifed that pt was unable to have stat mri's done due to not meeting stat criteria and it would have to be done in am. verbalized understanding.
Notes: labs drawn via peripheral stick x1 and sent to lab for stat admission orders.

NURSING PROCEDURE: OXYGEN THERAPY
PATIENT IDENTIFIER: Patient's identity verified by patient stating name, patient stating birth date, hospital ID bracelet.
OXYGEN THERAPY: Oxygen saturation 98%, by adult/pediatric oxisensor, single pulse oximetry reading, 2L oxygen given, via nasal cannula applied, Applied by via nasal cannula.
FOLLOW-UP: After procedure, oxygen saturation 99%.
SAFETY: Side rails up, Cart/Stretcher in lowest position, Family at bedside, Call light within reach, Hospital ID band on.

EKG INTERPRETATION
MONITOR STRIP: Monitor strip shows sinus tachycardia, with no ectopics.
12 LEAD EKG INTERPRETATION: Left bundle branch block.

NURSING ASSESSMENT: FOCUSED
CONSTITUTIONAL: History obtained from patient, Patient arrives, via Emergency Medical Services, Patient cooperative, Patient alert, Oriented to person, place and time, Skin warm, Skin dry, Mucous membranes pink, Patient is well-groomed, Patient complains of seizure like activity, **patient arrived via ems with c/o possible seizure activity that started about 1 month ago, and today patient began having episodes where she could not get air. periods of 10-15 seconds,.**
PAIN: **dull pain, back of head, on a scale 0-10 patient rates pain as 2, patient verbalized pain is worse after episodes.**
EYES: Focused eye assessment finding include pupils equally round and reactive to light, Left pupil 3 mm in size, Right pupil 3 mm in size.
NEURO: Focused neuro assessment findings include patient alert, cooperative, No facial droop noted, Speech coherent.
RESPIRATORY: Focused respiratory assessment findings include breath sounds clear, to the right upper lobe.
ABDOMEN: Focused abdominal assessment findings include abdomen soft.
MUSCULOSKELETAL: pedal pulse +3.
SAFETY: Side rails up, Cart/Stretcher in lowest position, Family at bedside, Call light within reach, Hospital ID band on.

Prepared: Mon Sep 19, 2016 10:20 by Interface Page: 10 of 11
SEE CHART IN ED PULSECHECK APPLICATION ARCHIVE FOR CHART ENTRY DATES AND TIMES.

Figure 7.[2]

As you can see from the second record, the physician can easily find what is important and what needs to be done to take the best possible care of the patient. Getting practicing physicians involved in the development and use of the electronic medical record (EMR) will make all the difference in helping physicians care for their patients instead of being a hindrance. So far, we are not achieving the goal of sharing information effectively, which was the initial impetus for the development of the electronic medical record. When we are able to easily share records, we will not only see patient care improve, but we will also see the cost of care go down. This is our goal as physicians, because we care deeply about giving each patient the best care possible and conserving capital so the whole population can be cared for effectively and efficiently.

WHOSE JOB IS IT ANYWAY?

As the practice of medicine has become more specialized and more divided between outpatient and inpatient care, the number of patient handoffs and care transitions has increased. Physicians transition care many times a day, yet we are notoriously bad at the process. We give too much information, or we give too little information, and sometimes we give no information at all. We expect patients to remember what was done to them in an environment that is foreign and stressful to them and extremely hard for them to understand. We do not address the problem list or keep up with medication reconciliation, and we wonder why that information isn't passed along. We rely on other people to do our work, and many times we place the burden of communicating information on staff that are neither trained nor qualified to do the job that is actually required of the physician. As physicians, despite all the roadblocks placed upon us, we must be sure that we communicate the information needed for transitions of care so our patients get the best care possible. The steps to how we can improve care with better communication are addressed in the following section. If we fulfill our duty, then we can make sure the information the receiving physician gets is the information they need.

GUIDELINES FOR COMMUNICATION

Recognizing the need for better communication is the first step towards starting to solve the problem. Going forward, we must standardize communication methods and hold accountable our physicians and staff to be sure communication is being done the right way at the right time in order to provide the best possible care for our patients. Physicians must understand the importance of quickly transferring accurate information in order to get the best patient outcome.

Far from being a bother to a physician, the referring physician calling the receiving doctor and explaining the care already provided and the work still needing to be done is the best way to be sure an accurate handoff has occurred. While a phone call is not always necessary, it can be the quickest and most accurate way to get the message delivered.

When setting up patient discharge programs, involving physicians early and finding the most effective means of communication based on physician preference, time sensitivity and information complexity is essential. We may need to use multiple means of communication to ensure necessary information has been sent and received accurately. Wading through a lengthy text message may not be the most effective way to communicate critical information. Consider protected emails, facsimiles, letters, calls, and when possible, direct access to the medical records. Remember, if one type of communication doesn't work, try another.

Consider the time of day and what the other physician might be doing. During early morning rounds, a text may work best. A call at lunch or after office hours may be better still. If your first try doesn't work, try changing your method. Doing the same thing over and over in the same way will not complete the task.

Above all, when inaccurate or incomplete transmission of information can directly lead to patient harm, the best way to deliver that information is by direct face-to-face or verbal communication between physicians or between physician and staff. If we keep in mind how we would like the information transferred if the patient were a member of our own family being treated, then we can begin to be consistently successful.

Going Forward

Getting it right is a fairly simple process, but the pressures of time and the explosion of medical knowledge as well as the multitude of ways to communicate has complicated the matter. So let's get back to the basics. In order to provide the best care possible, we must work as a team. We must share necessary information to be sure the patient is not only unharmed, but in fact has the best possible outcome given their medical condition. We must navigate the clutter, improve patient handoffs, and persist in getting the right information about the right patient at the right time to the right place in order to practice the best medicine possible.

This means generating a simple, accurate electronic medical record allowing each team member to completely fulfill his or her obligation to the patient. Information shared between providers needs to be understandable, accurate, and protected. We can use different types of communication depending on the situation and desired outcome.

Each physician must do the WHOLE job. As physicians in training, we are taught to evaluate the patient, come up with a diagnosis, and treat them accordingly. Somehow, we get the idea that completing the medical records in a timely manner is not part of the WHOLE job. However, no information can be transmitted, prescriptions filled or patients billed until the medical record is completed. So as physicians, we are responsible not only for treating the patient, but also for completing the paperwork. While it may seem easier to put that off, not completing the patient's record at the time keeps us from fully achieving the goal of great patient care.

TWELVE STEPS TO BETTER COMMUNICATION

I believe the following twelve steps will enhance better communication and improve patient outcomes.

1. *Keep it simple.* Let's simplify the way physicians interact with the EMR, allowing physicians to make medical decisions and not be data entry clerks.

2. *Summarize.* At the end of each patient encounter, make sure the EMR has an easily recognizable synopsis which outlines what was done and what should be done going forward.

3. *Say the right thing in the right way at the right time.* Give an accurate and complete transfer of care – a complete handoff. This can be done electronically, but if the patient's condition is complicated, the information should be communicated directly, physician to physician.

4. *Learn to use the tools.* Make the best use of software so accurate medication reconciliation and the problem list are done and completed with each encounter. Use software to develop timely and accurate physician notification of test results and changes in the patient's condition.

5. *Ensure everybody does his or her part.* Encourage each team member to do their part of patient care completely so

no one has to handle anyone else's responsibilities.

6. Know your options. Standardize communication between physicians and staff. Monitor and reassess the complete list of communication options, and hold each team member accountable for meeting them.

7. Close the loop. Be sure the message is not only sent, but also received. When there is the possibility of direct patient harm, communicate verbally, physician to physician and physician to staff. Keep in mind time-sensitive reports so the message is communicated quickly to avoid patient harm.

8. Verify – don't assume. Remember all forms of communication can lead to errors. Never assume, and always verify information.

9. Third time's a charm. If it takes more than three emails to get the information across, pick up the phone.

10. Direct is best. Remember the best way to communicate information is by talking directly to the other party and making sure the information is received and understood.

11. Know your audience. Practicing medicine is demanding and difficult, and trying to practice in a vacuum is impossible. Physicians need to take the time to get to know each other and understand each other. Hospitalists should know their referring primary care doctors. Specialists should know their referring doctors. Medicine is a team sport, and each player must give his or her best effort.

12. It doesn't begin or end with you. Understand patient care doesn't start and end with your part of the care. The best medical care is a continuum, one physician to another and to the larger team as well, so good quality documentation and information transfer is what is best for each patient.

* * * * *

So as we close our discussion on communication and the need for improvement, let's celebrate the little wins we see every day when someone writes a perfect note or a fellow physician calls with information you need for a patient or when a fellow physician answers your page at two in the morning. Remember, none of us practices in a vacuum, and we must share our thoughts and concerns. If we do, we will be better physicians for it and our patients will receive the care they need and deserve.

Epilogue

THROUGHOUT THIS BOOK, we have examined the problems poor communication between doctors and healthcare providers can cause. We have also explored the bewildering array of ways to communicate medical information in this age of the electronic medical record. Many studies have shown how the electronic medical record has slowed physicians at work and how new ways of communications may not necessarily lead to better health outcomes.[1] As we move forward in our profession, we must consider the possibility that our biggest problem may be the interface between the physician and the electronic health record, leading to the loss of true communication between the physician and the patient.

Desperate Times Call for Desperate Measures

First, we should throw out the keyboard. The physician should not be put in the position of having to pay more attention to typing then to hearing what the patient has to say. There should be nothing between the patient and the physician, and certainly not a keyboard. We must change the interface so that physicians can concentrate on the patient and allow for true communication to occur.

With the new voice recognition programs and our ability to instantly communicate over video, we should not have to type or check boxes to record the interaction between patient and physician. Telemedicine facilitates instant communication with subspecialists in rural areas and has made it possible for patients to get care wherever they live. Let's discuss what a possible future scenario looks like when we take advantage of all of the electronic communication available to us with the endpoint being better direct patient-to-physician communication.

The Medical Visit Simplified

In the future of healthcare and especially primary care, we should be able to improve the interaction between physician and patient and take advantage of all of the possibilities allowed by new modes of electronic communication. The example below shows an example of a patient visiting a physician and the remarkable opportunities we have to make it work better and improve patient care.

* * * * *

Ms. Parker has an appointment with her doctor Dr. Belk. She comes to the office and checks in by using a code supplied by the office on her cellphone. Since Ms. Parker is an established patient, her medical information has already been updated in the computer and she does not have to interact with the receptionist, who knows that she is checked in and that her information is correct. When the exam room is available, Ms. Parker is taken to it by a medical assistant. The exam room has no computer keyboard. There is only a large Smart Board monitor present on the wall.

The medical assistant talks to the Smart Board, records Ms. Parker's vital signs, and notes changes in her review of systems or medications. She also records any interaction with other providers that has occurred since Ms. Parker's last visit. Ms. Parker can also interact with the Smart Board and look at her lab work from her last visit as well as the results of any other studies that have been performed.

When Dr. Belk enters the room, he or she notifies the Smart Board so it recognizes the doctor's voice and their interaction can occur. While talking to Ms. Parker, the information is recorded on the Smart Board and into the medical record by the voice-activated system. Again, there is no keyboard in the room. This allows Dr. Belk to actually talk directly to Ms. Parker to examine the patient and record information in real time. Dr. Belk can also review lab work, radiology images, and other information about the patient by using the Smart Board. In addition, Ms. Parker's medication can be reviewed and adjusted as needed.

On her visit today, Ms. Parker has a concern about her ongoing treatment for pancreatic cancer. In order to get a rapid response to her questions, Dr. Belk connects instantly with her oncologist, Dr. Redmond, over the Smart Board. They then have a conversation involving both physicians and Ms. Parker to determine her next steps in her plan of treatment. This is also recorded into the medical record, avoiding an unnecessary trip to the oncologist office, and clearly documenting the plan of care for all parties.

Finally Dr. Belk finishes the examination, dictates a plan of treatment, and orders prescriptions over the Smart Board. Those prescriptions are sent directly to Ms. Parker's pharmacy. A follow-up appointment is scheduled and Dr. Belk leaves the room and finalizes the plan of treatment in a short, easily understood paragraph that other physicians can see in the record. The medical assistant returns to the room and using the Smart Board, shows Ms. Parker educational videos addressing her concerns. The checkout is easy and the data is immediately updated in the record, which can then be shared with other physicians who care for Ms. Parker.

* * * * *

To summarize, it seems to me that when it comes to physician-to-physician communication, we're getting things backward. Rather than focusing on the tool, program, application, device or system that promises to be the answer to all our communication challenges, our goal of an ongoing profession-wide commitment to successful communication should determine how we select both our approach (our model) and the tools we use to achieve it. That goal, and our commitment to it, will illuminate the way forward in our constantly-changing field.

Notes

Chapter One:
[1]CRICO Strategies, http://www.rmfstrategies.com
[2]Melissa Bailey, February 1, 2016, www.statnews.com, Communication failures linked to 1,744 deaths in five years, US malpractice study finds
[3]Estimate by the Joint Chief, http://www.jointcommission.org/assets/1/6/tst_hoc_persp_08_12.pdf
[4]Figure 1. Source: www.cloud.spok.com/EB-AMER-Joint-Commission-Goal-2.pdf
[5]Spok.com, A Guide to the Joint Commission's Communication Goal, page 3
[6]Spok.com, A Guide to the Joint Commission's Communication Goal, page 3
[7]www.merriam-webster.com/dictionary/professionalism
[8] www.annenbergclassroom.org/Files/Documents/Timelines/HealthCare.pdf

Chapter Two:
[1]Figure 2. Source: Spok.com, A Guide to the Joint Commission's Communication Goal, page 2.

Chapter Three:
[1]The Untold Secret: How Poor Communication Leads to Medical Malpractice, Dr. Zeev Kain, http://drzeevkain.health/the-untold-secret-how-poor-communication-leads-to-medical-malpractice/
[2]Khanna R, Wachsberg K, Marouni A, Feinglass J, Williams MV, Wayne DB, Night or Weekend Admission and Outcomes. J. Hosp. Med 2011;1;10-14. doi:10.1002/jhm.833
[3]https://www.psqh.com/analysis/nurse-to-physician-communications-connecting-for-safety/
[4]https://www.ncbi.nlm.nih.gov/books/NBK2649/
[5]https://www.ncbi.nlm.nih.gov/books/NBK2649/
[6] https://www.ncbi.nlm.nih.gov/books/NBK2649/
[7]Figure 3. Source: Amy Keller, April 26, 2016 https://dailynurse.com/how-to-talk-to-doctors/
[8]https://www.psqh.com/analysis/nurse-to-physician-communications-connecting-for-safety/

Chapter Four:
[1]a study funded by the Agency for Healthcare Research and Quality (AHRQ) and published in the February 3, 2009, issue of the Annals of Internal Medicine.

Chapter Five:
[1] www.pcpcc.org/about/medical-home
[2]www.aha.org/advocacy/current-and-emerging-payment-models/pfsmacraqpp
[3] Tamblyn R, Eguale T, Huang A, Winslade N, Doran P. The Incidence and

Determinants of Primary Nonadherence With Prescribed Medication in Primary Care: A Cohort Study. Ann Intern Med. 2014;160:441-450. doi: 10.7326/M13-1705

Chapter Six:
[1] www.practicefusion.com/what-is-meaningful-use/
[2] www.pressganey.com/resources/program-summary/frequently-asked-questions-about-hcahps
[3] www.modernhealthcare.com/article/20170828/SPONSORED/170829897

Chapter Seven:
[1] http://www.mayoclinicproceedings.org/article/S0025-6196(15)00716-8/abstract
[2] The Untold Secret: How Poor Communication Leads to Medical Malpractice, Dr. Zeev Kain, http://drzeevkain.health/the-untold-secret-how-poor-communication-leads-to-medical-malpractice/
[3] Rand Health Quarterly, V 3(4), Winter 2014. "Factors Affecting Physician Professional Satisfaction and Their Implications for Patient Care, Health Systems, and Health Policy." ©2014 Rand Corporation.
[4] searchhealthit.techtarget.com/definition/meaningful-use-stage-3

Chapter Eight:
[1] Epstein RM, Hundert EM. Defining and Assessing Professional Competence. *JAMA*. 2002;287(2):226-235. doi:10.1001/jama.287.2.226
[2] The Untold Secret: How Poor Communication Leads to Medical Malpractice, Dr. Zeev Kain, http://drzeevkain.health/the-untold-secret-how-poor-communication-leads-to-medical-malpractice/
[3] Figure 4. Source: www.medicalrepublic.com/au/doctor-cant-read-writing/10370
[4] Figure 5. Source: https://media.springernature.com/full/springer-static/image/art%3A10.1186%2F1472-6963-11-199/MediaObjects/12913_2010_Article_1730_Fig2_HTML.jpg
[5] www.haponline.org/Newsroom/Media/HIPAA-Guidelines
[6] www.healthcareitnews.com/news/10-largest-hipaa-breaches-2012

Chapter Nine:
[1] Figure 6. Source: Dr. Irvin's personal notes
[2] Figure 7. Source: Dr. Irvin's personal notes

Epilogue:
[1] www.ajmc.com/journals/issue/2013/2013-11-vol19-sp/the-impact-of-electronic-health-record-use-on-physician-productivity

Acknowledgments

Like most people, my life's experience is made up of interactions with and influences from others with whom I have been fortunate to make contact. There have been good and bad experiences, but I always learned from each and every encounter.

Over the years I have benefited from watching the work of many great physicians and administrators who cared deeply about patient care and improving the process of care delivery. I am blessed to have known and learned from them.

Lastly, I want to acknowledge the help of Deb Burdick, who guided me through the writing process and helped me complete this book.

About the Author

AS A PRACTICING family physician and Chief Medical Officer for over 40 years, Dr. Irvin has lived the book he's written. His undergraduate degree in business management from Mississippi State University gave him a different perspective when he attended medical school. Dr. Irvin is a graduate of the University of Mississippi Medical School and completed his Internship and Residency programs at Sacred Heart Hospital in Pensacola, Florida. His interest in lack of communication between physicians accelerated after a patient suffered a poor outcome due to a failure to communicate a test result in a timely manner. Dr. Irvin earned an MBA and has spent the last several years working to help improve patient care and physician hospital alignment.

Made in United States
Orlando, FL
30 January 2024